A donation to Stroke Research & Rehabilitation from every Sale

No Regrets, No Surrender!
By Roger Turner

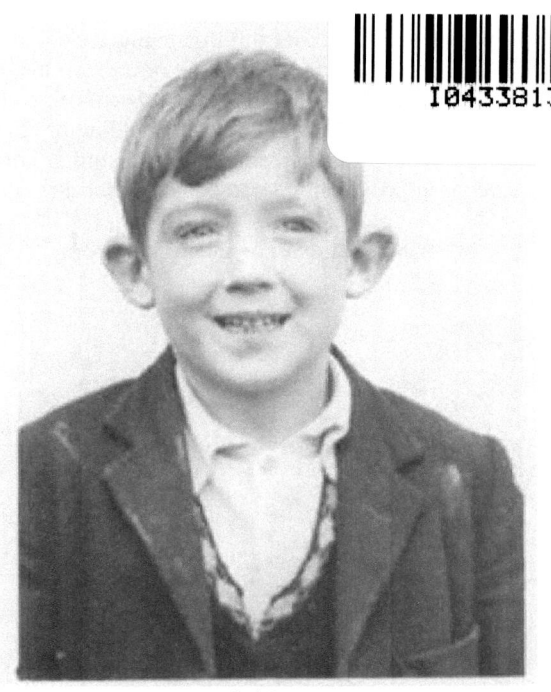

aged 10 years.
A Story of a Stroke Survivor!

Published by New Generation Publishing in 2016

Copyright © Roger Turner 2016

First Edition

The author asserts the moral right under the Copyright, Designs and Patents Act 1988 to be identified as the author of this work.

All Rights reserved. No part of this publication may be reproduced, stored in a retrieval system or transmitted, in any form or by any means without the prior consent of the author, nor be otherwise circulated in any form of binding or cover other than that which it is published and without a similar condition being imposed on the subsequent purchaser.

www.newgeneration-publishing.com

 New Generation Publishing

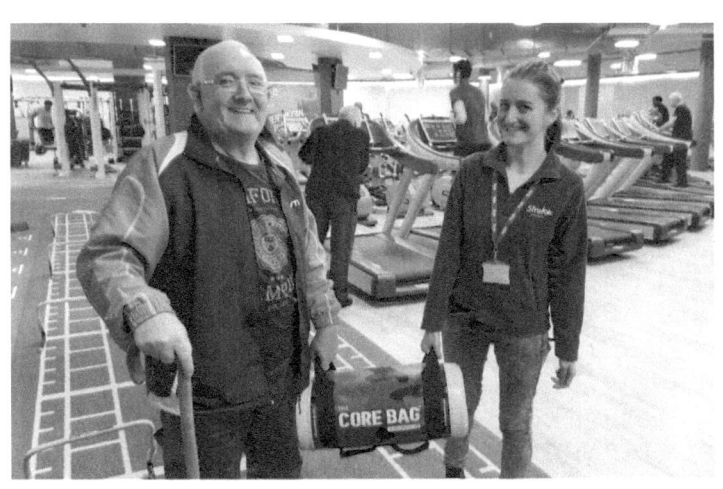

At Pond's Forge Gym with Volunteer Helper Rebecca

Contents

PREFACE 1
Foreword 2
PART 1 - Icmeler, Turkey 5
  CHAPTER 1/ Icmeler, Turkey 5
  CHAPTER 2 / Ahu Hospital, Turkey 8
  CHAPTER 3 / The Insurance Doctor Arrives 18
  CHAPTER 4 / Welcome to the UK 21
  CHAPTER 5 / Lung Problems 28
  CHAPTER 6 / 1st UK Physiotherapy 31
  CHAPTER 7/ Rehabilitation Centre. 36
  CHAPTER 8 / Room 15 43
PART 2 54
  CHAPTER 9 / Going Home 54
  CHAPTER 10/ 1st Stair Lift Ride 62
  CHAPTER 11 / Standing Ovation 71
  CHAPTER 12 / New Gates 76
  CHAPTER 13 / F.E.S. 92
  CHAPTER 14 / Driver Assessment Day 97
  CHAPTER 15 / Hyper Baric Chamber 101
  CHAPTER 16 / Pond's Forge Gym 105
  CHAPTER 17 / Benidorm 117
  CHAPTER 18 / Crossfit Gym 126
  CHAPTER 19 / Flat Tyre 135
  CHAPTER 20 / Scooter Test 141
  CHAPTER 21 / The Jolly Season 143
  CHAPTER 22 / 2016 146
  CHAPTER 23 / Emotions and Feelings 149
  CHAPTER 24 / Stroke Recovery 152
  MY FALLS & STUMBLES 154
  CASE HISTORIES 156
ABOUT THE AUTHOR: 170
MY HEROES 177

SPECIAL ACKNOWLEDGEMENTS 179
PLACES THAT I HAVE VISITED AND SITES
THAT I HAVE SEEN 181
A FOOTNOTE 183

PREFACE

I am writing my Story in the hope that it will help other Stroke survivors, who find themselves in the same boat as me and to realize that it's not only them that has had such a horrid time. Many people are devastated by strokes and have to accept major changes in their lives & not just to them, but their entire support team as well............
Good Luck everybody!

FOREWORD

BY
EMMA RICHARDS.MSC. MACP. HCPC. GRAD DIP.
Neuro physiotherapist

It has been a privilege and a real pleasure working with Roger. He is, in the true sense of the word a survivor who has turned his rehabilitation into his road to recovery. He has taught me so much Roger needed empowering to take control back of his life; he needed to find ways of progressing himself.

Roger is a resilient, some might call stubborn! Man from Sheffield who wants to share his experiences and how he empowered himself on his road to recovery. He has a strong sense of "what's right and what's wrong" with the strength of steel balanced against such fairness; he doesn't feel pain "I'm a Yorkshireman".

So often with all the current austerity measures and the restraints in our wonderful National Health service; rehabilitation therapists feel it necessary to instil a sense of reality into their patients, suggesting that recovery is often limited this can lead them to focus on managing the disability rather than empowering the stroke survivor to focus on what they can do and believe that things are still possible.

What they really mean is, there will be limitations within how much the rehabilitation service can offer them but shouldn't mean they give up expecting to achieve further recovery, this can and will continue for the rest of their lives.

This inspirational story will help those who have suffered a Stroke to know, that there is hope, and that the road to recovery is long but "keep going" and focus what you're achieving.

E.Richards@shu.ac.uk

This book is Dedicated to my Loving Wife

Maureen Turner xxx

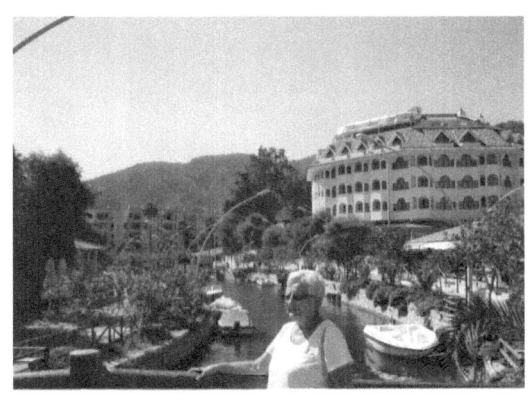

PART 1
ICMELER, TURKEY

CHAPTER 1/ Day 1

Saturday 21st June 2014

The sun was high in the sky on this cloudless day. My wife Maureen, and I decided to go for a morning stroll around the village. We called for a spot of lunch at *Tin Tin's* bar /restaurant. I ordered a pint of Shandy for myself and a small bottle of water for Maureen from Mustafa, one of the owners. We ordered the special Chicken fried rice, a favourite of ours.

Once the eating and the people watching were over, we walked the 300 yards back to our Hotel, the Kapmar, where we had one week left of our three weeks holiday.

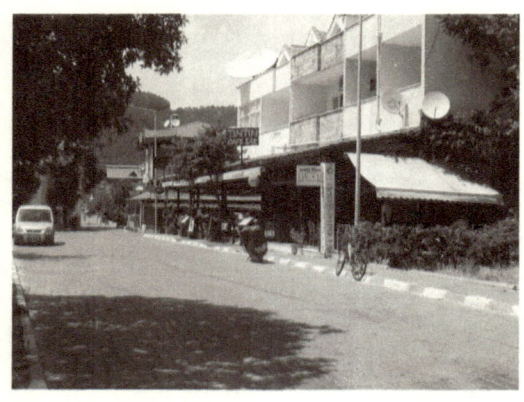

Upon arrival at the Hotel, Maureen, who was wearing her swimming costume under her shorts and top, said that she was going to the pool for a spot of sunbathing and a swim. I told here that I would pop up to our room and get <u>*changed*</u>, in to my swim shorts. Boy was that an understatement and one that would change our lives, <u>probably</u> forever!.

I went into our bathroom to discharge the shandy. At this point I started having a stroke I thought to myself is this just a T.I.A. or a full one for real this time! But alas it was for real and the nightmare of all nightmares was beginning. I thought I had better make my way, as best I can, into the bedroom as quickly as possible! I recognized the symptoms as I had had a TIA, a mini-stroke, 5 years earlier. I just about managed to fling myself onto the bed before the full impact of the stroke hit me.

With my right hand I managed to grab hold of the room phone to signal down to reception, or so I thought! Unfortunately no one answered. I then started to shout for help, but no one could have heard me, as help was not forthcoming. I think that upon reflection, this shouting kept me both fully awake during this whole stroke process and more importantly kept the brain fully functioning

I waited ....!

After a further half hour my wife arrived to find out, whether I was going to have a swim or was I having a nap instead. As soon as she saw me, she swung into action. She did not panic at all, which is just what was needed, and something that made me extremely proud of her. Maureen could not raise anyone on the phone either, so she had to go down from our *top floor room* to reception to ask for medical help. (Apparently the internal phone system was currently out of action but the outside lines worked.) Mehmet the concierge rang for this help immediately!

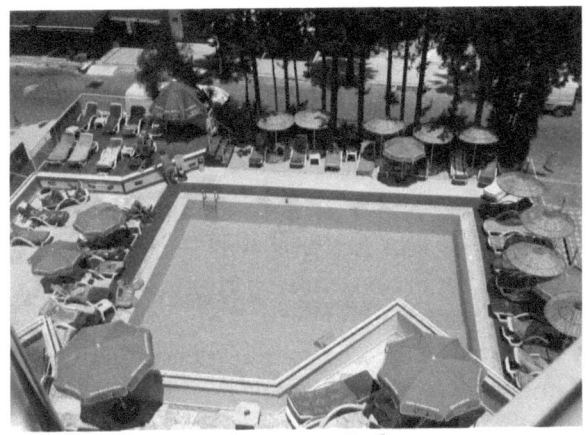

View from our Balcony

The Paramedics arrived within minutes assessed the situation very quickly told my wife to bring the Insurance documents & passports etc with us. They bungled me up and put me on a transfer chair for transportation, first down in the lift to the reception area and then off to the Hospital.

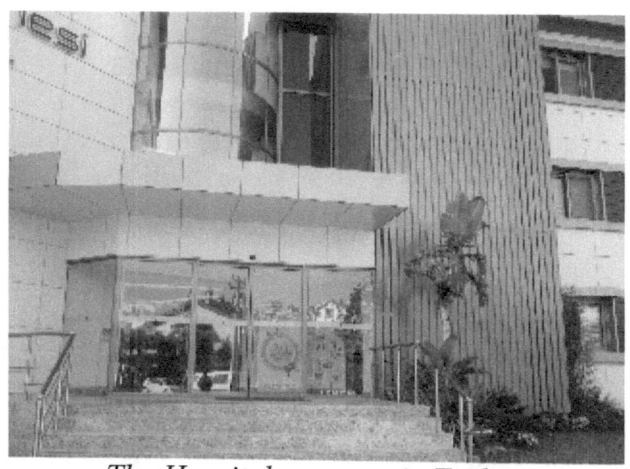

The Hospital entrance in Turkey.

CHAPTER 2 / Day 1
THE HOSPITAL

"Ahu Hastanesi" a Tourist/Holidaymakers Hospital in the Mugla area, and was only about 5/6 miles away from the Hotel. This hospital was, as it name implies, brand new. The Paramedics en-route and the Hospital professionals upon arrival saved my life.

I was taken to the emergency department for a full Assessment. It was then that I had the first of my cranial MRI scans. Thereafter I was taken to ICU where I was attached to various machines to monitor and drug me.

The MRI scan confirmed to the medical team the severity of my haemorrhagic stroke. A bleed, inside my brain, which is considered pretty much a very dangerous place to have one, being much more severe then on the outer side of the brain, or by an arterial blockage, caused by a pieces of floating cholesterol, which had formed into plaque and obstructed the blood flow to my brain via the Carotid Arteries.(An Ischemic attack) They found that my Liver was not working 100%, so they put me on some medication to sort it, which it did, but it took a week for it to fully stabilize. They never did find out what had caused the Liver irregularity in the first place, so maybe it was just the stroke or too many G & T's. Unfortunately we shall never know!

Without my wife, and being in Hospital in a Sunni dominated Muslim Country with their different Language, customs, habits and Religious tolerances etc, would have been just too frightening for the brain to contemplate, let alone feeling very vulnerable. Thank goodness that my Maureen was there to love and protect me, from all these influences, be they real or unreal. You know it was just a fear of the unknown and what was to happen to me!

I was in the hospital in Turkey for fifteen long days, during that time I received a minimal amount of physiotherapy. This took place in my bed in ICU, where I stayed for 11 or 12 days until another scan proved that the bleed had stopped and my brain was in no further danger.

The following day the Staff brought me, what I can only describe as an open fronted Plastic Wellington. I did not know this at the time, but the Hospital was actually trying to prevent me from having "Drop Foot" this practice was never carried out once back in the UK and I have a dropped foot today. Whether the Plastic Wellington would have prevented my foot from dropping or not, we shall never know for sure, but we can speculate. The UK hospital and Rehab units both told me at a later date that this would correct itself once I was up and walking! **Still waiting!**

I had struggled for about 8/9 days without needing a bed pan. It was decided to help nature along with the use of a round bottle full of what looked like soapy water. The bottle had a round 3 or 4 inches long spout in the top through which the fluid would flow to assist my colon to do its stuff. It took all of 10 minutes to help Vesuvius erupt, in actual fact it was more of a Mount St. Helens blowing its top than a gentle versuvian eruption. I felt a lot happier after that episode which I would not be repeating in a hurry!

A ward orderly actually carried me from ICU to the ward, no mean feat as I arrived at the Hospital weighing about 16 stones 3 pounds. This new hospital did not have any form of hoist or lifting equipment to move patients from one place to another or to just lift them out of bed onto a trolley or commode or whatever! The poor Orderlies' had to do it every time muscles were needed! *Better than a Gym "body-attack" workout any time*.

On my 3rd night in ICU, there was such a commotion! *"All visitors must leave and wait outside"* was the command. Why what up? I asked…No answer, nobody spoke English or not enough to be able to explain the reason(s). It turned out there was a lady from Belgium in the next bed, on which they performed emergency open-chest surgery, in situ! Amazing! Apparently there was no time to move her as she was in a very serious condition. The surgeon was successful with this emergency surgery and saved the woman's life! What was even more amazing, she was later taken by Helicopter to the Airport for onward repatriation to Brussels.(I hope she got there in a reasonable condition, that is alive!) Whilst all this was going on, I was in complete limbo as was my wife, who was now downstairs in the café wondering what on earth was happening up on the Ward. We found out much later of the emergency and the procedures needed to save her life and of the surgeons heroics. My wife was eventually allowed back in to see me after about a 90mins break, much to my relief, as I was very worried as to what had happened to her.

Starting the following morning they began checking on my breathing capacity, by the use of a series of connecting tubes with balls in the bottom of these tubes. Sometimes I was told to blow the balls to the top of this piece of equipment and at other times, to suck them to the top, this was a lot harder, but with determination, I succeeded! We did this check every day for 4 days.

On my 9th day, Granddaughter Annabell and her boyfriend Ryan, who had just arrived, for their annual holidays, came to see me. Poor Annabell was distraught at seeing the state of me as was Ryan. After a little chat and an update on my health and progress, they felt a lot happier. They told me that they had been brought to the hospital by some friends of ours, these friends were waiting outside the ward to come and see me, when they got the go ahead to do so. The two friends, Muzzy and Ibo, who both worked in our favourite watering-hole, asked if they too could come and visit me also, so that they could report back to the other staff we know in the bar. It was great to see all four of my visitors, if only for a short while. One can tire very easily after a Stroke.

A couple of days later, Vince, the owner of a bar/restaurant/apartment block, we had stayed at on many occasions over the years, also called to see me and has continued to keep in touch by email ever since. This guy is amazing! He helped my wife with all of her problems, and there were many. He has been a great friend of ours for many years and many more to come, I am sure of that!

One day I had a Chest x-ray in my bed. The imaging specialist arrived with all the equipment and a fully lead lined overall for protection from the rays, which must only be active on his side of the equipment as I had no protection. The result of such was that I did not have any heart or chest problems ……..Oh goodie!

More good news came later when they served me half a banana after my evening meal. *Yippee!* *Some soup, half banana or the occasional ice cream helped me to survive the comestible challenge*, this challenge appears to be pretty standard in hospitals the world over and which in itself helped me to lose 2 stones 4 pounds, during my stay with them. *Yippee again!* This was good for my figure but not necessarily for my strength, which I would certainly need as time progressed along with my initial internal recovery. I received a final x-ray whilst in their care, this third one gave me the all-clear to travel home. *About time too!*. Believe me two weeks and one day in a foreign hospital, that does things slightly different from us Brits and who generally don't speak any English to explain what or why is quite frustrating, to say the least. Don't get me wrong, there were 3 Interpreters, but the Hospital was full of non-Turkish speaking patients, so there were just not enough of these interpreters to go around. They were in great demand, especially from us Non-International Speaking brits!

My wonderful Wife who had the most horrendous time with "my little problem", plus sorting the Insurance out and having to pack up the cases, when we were ready to fly home was absolutely amazing,

I could never thank or love her enough. She was kept sane thanks to the wives of two of the other English patients, also there with their little problems.

These ladies, Pam & Gloria used to help Maureen with getting buses to and fro between Hotel and Hospital and they would then meet up for an evening meal or a glass of wine etc, before turning in for the day. They also popped in to see me and help keep my chin up that first week.

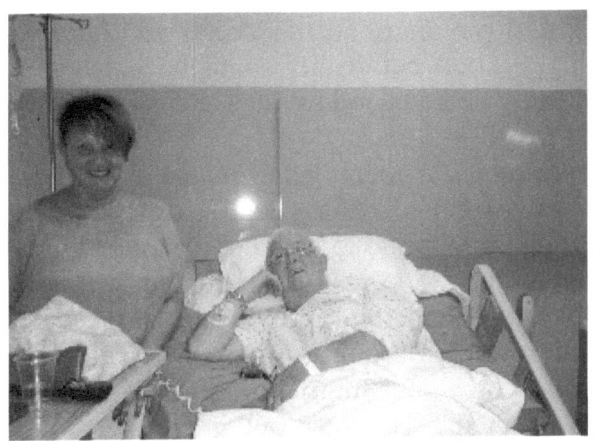

Me and Denise in the ICU Dept .in the Hospital.

That is until the cavalry, in the form of daughter Denise, arrived. She stayed with my wife and supported her and me immensely during her time with us. Denise came for 10 days and was still there for a couple of days, after we were allowed to fly home.

We are still in contact with Pam & Gloria, who have both been back on Holiday with their husbands a few times since they got back home. Pam's husband Anton had slipped in their hotel bathroom and hit his head on the tiled floor this had caused him to have a mini-Stroke.

Fortunately, if you can call it that, it was not as severe as my Stroke and he was allowed to leave on the 3rd July. Whereas Gloria's husband Paul, had a heart condition which was treated but was always declare everything to the Medical Insurance people. If we hadn't, we estimate that our Bill would have been at least £80000, not worth the hassle, is it! allowed home after 14 days, only 10 of which, was when we were there. They had had Health Insurance problems! Apparently Paul had not fully declared all medical issues and was therefore told he would have to pay roughly £10000 before he would be allowed home. Fortunately he had good savings and could do this. A lesson for ALL,

One evening a young lad of nineteen was admitted with stab wounds. His young lady had bought a blouse that was found to be faulty when they got back to their Hotel. Next day they returned to the shop to ask for a replacement or refund. The shopkeeper took exception to their request as he considered, probably through is own poor translation, that his honesty was being insulted. He took out a knife and stabbed young Kevin, twice in the stomach. Kevin was a fit guy, and with his family, who flew out immediately to help him, recovered and was allowed to fly home 6 days later. On our pen-ultimate day another stabbing occurred in the local town, a bar fight! This young man had only superficial wounds, so was quickly patched up and sent on his way.

Day10. What a relief the Medical Insurance clearance came through.
Phew! We can breathe again.

Especially Maureen who had been under enormous pressure until it arrived and still tons more pressure forever, worrying! Until you have been in this situation, you cannot realize just how heart stopping it must feel before the nod comes through to Proceed with full backing.

**Hospital Summary:
They saved my life!**

- They gave me some Physiotherapy, (about 3 sessions): The physiotherapist lady repeatedly said, when one tried to do any movement….. "shlowly! shlowly!

- They also daily fitted an open fronted, sort of wellington, to my affected left leg, for a few hours at a time. This was to help prevent drop foot occurring, and maybe if they had carried this on with this in the UK, it would not have happened. However, it did and over a year and a half later, I still this problem, but we are still trying to activate the affected muscles and will continue to do so.

- I was taken by wheelchair to the day room area for chats and looks outside, on two occasions (Bliss! as it is really nice to get an idea of where you are and what the area around you looks

like) The staff swung my legs over to and down the right-hand side of my bed, sat me upright, picked me up and literally just dropped me in the wheelchair.
- (or at least that is what it felt like to me)

- They sorted my Liver out.

- Unintentionally they helped me lose weight, a really good thing. (Two stones five pounds in total)

- They cancelled all of the tablets that I had been previously taking daily, i.e. Statins, Aspirins' Allopurinol and Ramipril.

- <u>Statins</u> to control my cholesterol level.

- <u>Aspirin</u> to keep my blood a little thinner and act as an anti-clotting agent.

- <u>Ramipril</u> to regulate my Blood Pressure.

Three three drugs were supposed to help stop me having a Stroke,
One thinks that they failed badly! But maybe I would have been worse off without these!

- <u>Allopurinol</u> to keep control of my Uric Acid production, and help alleviate problems associated with the Gout that I had had for at least 20years "I no longer have Gout". ***What a Bonus and what an extreme way to get rid of it!***

- They put me on an epilepsy drug, "just in case?" This was withdrawn by the Royal Hallamshire Hospital when I got back to the UK,

Whilst in the Turkish hospital I received various family phone calls, these were gratefully received. It really takes you back to reality and a sense of being part of the UK once more, when you get to talk to family back at HOME.

CHAPTER 3 / Day 13

Thursday 3rd July 2014

THE INSURANCE COMPANY DOCTOR, ARRIVED

A Doctor Gareth from the Medical Insurance Company arrived to take charge of getting us back to good old Sheffield. This was not an easy task for him as he had to find flights that could accommodate me on a stretcher. Apparently not many airlines have the right type of seats which fold down and can accommodate stretchers. Plus seats for Maureen and Gareth and all his medical gear, plus the attendant transfer paperwork that would be needed. We had to pay for 10 seats on the aircrafts, to be able to transport us back to the UK. He sorted my onwards drugs package and obtained copies of all the medical records and x-rays pertaining to me that needed to be transferred onto my new "Carers", back in England.

Gareth had been a Specialist in patient recovery from overseas accidents/emergencies for 24 years. He usually organized and controlled the recovery of two or three sick souls, each month. He epitomized professionalism in all aspects, and especially that of being able to give my wife the solid support and assurances that I am sure she needed.

Departure Day. Day 16
6th July 2014

Departure day began for Maureen and the doctor at about 05:00hrs and they arrived at the Ward by about 06:00hrs. There I was **starker's!** Ready to be sent back to the UK in all my glory, or not as some would say. Maureen had been told not to bother with any clothes for me, as I would have my Pyjamas on. *Alas no!*

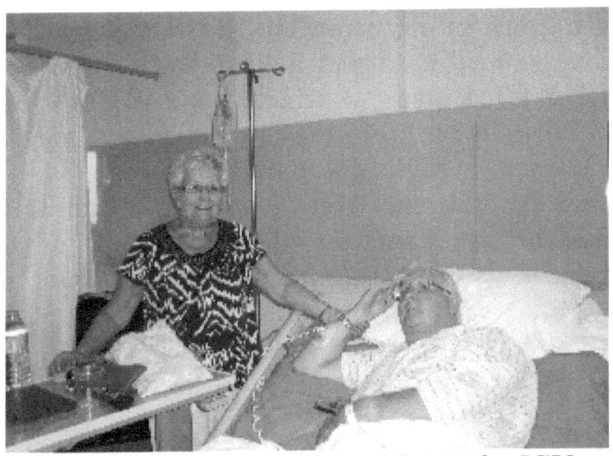

My wife Maureen and I, whilst in the ICU.

The hospital was not that generous, even at roughly £1000 per night plus food plus whatever else I may need such as x-ray's of various types and specialist Doctors and nursing staff. So with all my clothes packed in our cases in an anti-room downstairs at the hospital, she had to make arrangements to buy a pair of Pyjamas from the hospital for me to travel home in.

Maureen had trouble finding anyone from whom she could buy a pair, let alone someone who could speak English, eventually! she did find a receptionist who could help. After various tense and upsetting moments Maureen agreed to buy a pair for the cost of about £26. With this then sorted and me clad in my despatch suit, we were taken by private ambulance to Dalaman airport for the first leg of our Journey to Istanbul. The flight left Dalaman about 9:45 and arrived at Istanbul about one hour later. On arrival at Istanbul we were put in a Warehouse style of building to await our onward flight to Manchester. Lovely!

Carrying me, on my stretcher off the plane, was not an easy task. The Airport helpers had to wangle the stretcher 90 degrees to where some of the helpers were knelt in the aisle. My stretcher and me were placed on their backs and they had to crawl with me towards the exit and then on to the "hydraulic lift" vehicle to the terminal, where they left us in a warehouse style building for roughly 2.5 hours, with only a little water between all 3 of us.

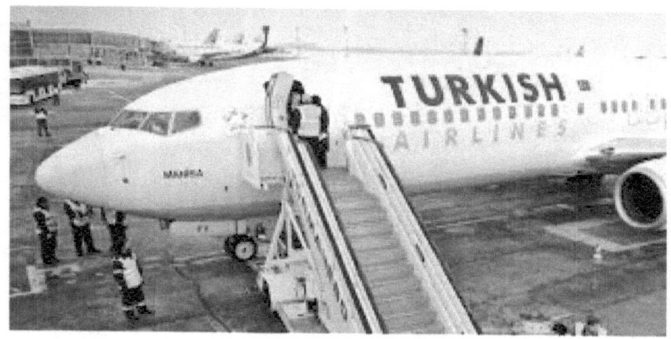

After which we were flown to Manchester without any further upset and where I was removed from the plane with a lot more aplomb and decorum. We arrived at 1540 hours where an Ambulance awaited us for the last leg of our journey to the Royal Hallamshire Hospital, Sheffield. U.K.

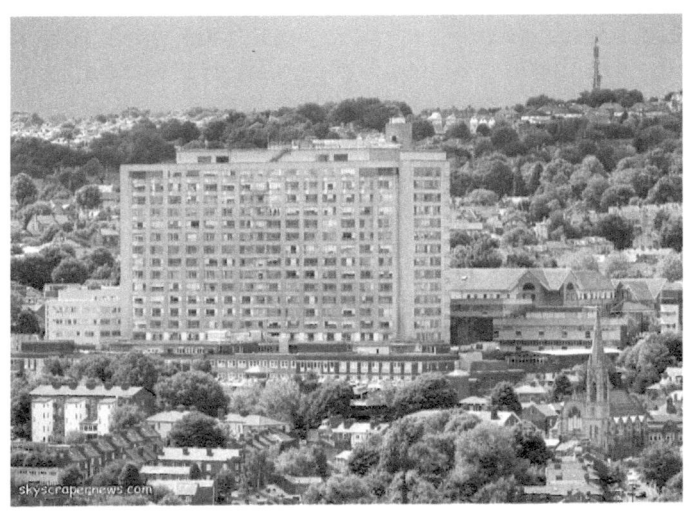

CHAPTER 4 / Day 16

6th July 2014

Welcome to the UK

This last leg of our journey home was horrendous. It was the day of the Tour de France, from Leeds to Sheffield. We had loads of detours on the way to Sheffield and when we got there lots of road closures and even more detours, the Ambulance driver, who was from Manchester area didn't have a clue as to how to get past all these diversions. With me lying flat in the back of his Ambulance I could not see much to help either. When we did manage to get to the hospital, we could not find a way in, road closures again! We had to drive around the place for half an hour or so, before luck won out!

We had made it in and were taken straight up to SAU1 a stroke assessment ward. God what a relief it was to have got to the "Royal Hallamshire", for us both. It must have been a massive relief to Maureen, to have got me back to Sheffield, *still alive*! I spent a couple of nights in SAU1 then transferred up to SU1, the specialist Stroke Floor.

I was put into a single bedded room. Room No.8. (Which I ought to tell you is now my unlucky number replacing the number13) My second night there was frightening. I starting feeling unwell and after about an hour, I projectile vomited! It was so violent that the contents of my stomach hit the wall 10/11 feet in front of me and then vertical in the bed a further 3 times.

If it wasn't for a patient in the next room who raised the alarm, I would have died there and then, in my bed. There was no patient buzzer, as it was broken! The "night nurse" eventually came running; "Oh my god" was the exclamation. She then spent the next 60 minutes or so cleaning me and every little bit of the bed and frame, as the mess had gone absolutely everywhere. No excuse or reason as to her not being more available was forthcoming the whole time that I was in the hospital.

The 14 broken patient buzzers were repaired, as if by Magic, the very next day. No other patient call buzzers to my knowledge, were broken again throughout the rest of my 5 weeks with them!

The following morning when my wife heard about what had happened, was the first time I realized that it is not a good idea to upset her. She rang up and went ballistic at the nursing staff and insisted that I be moved onto one of the wards with immediate effect. This was dealt with all haste as I was given a new home in bed D in ward 6 before 11o'clock as is when my wife arrived.

8th July   Day 18

The new "home" had 4 beds in it, Bed "A" had Abdul a remarkable cheery sort of guy, Bed "B" had Gerry a quiet English gentleman, and in Bed "C" was Eddie and lastly Bed "D" had me in it. We were all at different stages in our recovery. I being the last man to arrive on the ward was obviously in the worst condition out of the four of us.

Abdul had good upper body movement but was still not good at walking any more than 2 or 3 paces. Gerry too seemed pretty active, but a lot of this was just bluster, as he was a lot less capable, once scrutinized. Eddie, in Bed "C", was the typical happy go lucky Jamaican, who was overseen by his ever attentive ex-nurse wife, Marlene who was nearly always about, or so it seemed. The next few days were spent getting accustomed to the hospital regime and, of course, my new best friends Abdul, Gerry & Eddie.

The day started at about 0630hrs, when the first of the daytime nursing staff arrived. First job was the infamous bed bath, a time of great hilarity or not, as was the case. I.e. god this waters bloody freezing, must be the ice cubes, Nurse Hatchet would say, trying her best to wind you up. It usually worked! I don't know why because it was never cold.

However, the relief was so great when the water was released onto you. You then just ate out of her hand and did exactly as she asked or demanded in her usual jolly fashion.

After all four of us in the ward had been *sanitized*, a process that could last a couple of hours it was breakfast time! Various other Nurses or Student nurses would also have this opportunity to cleanse us. One of which was a Gay lad, he was funny, He used to pass me a flannel and say "Do you want to do your privates" **"Privates"** I would say "they young man have been **"Publics"** for weeks" Ha! Ha!

Breakfast came.....Have you ever tried to feed yourself, lying totally flat in bed with your rollaway table placed over your stomach area but about 9inches over it, with a bowl of cereal and a cup of tea on it, NO! Well I'll tell you, the cereal you get everywhere, with some actually entering your mouth. Goodie! It would be better if staff could just spend a little time assisting you, but with the NHS funding cuts, it was just not possible, As for the tea, you have to wait whilst it cools, so as not to scold yourself. Later you get to sit up a little and have a bit of a chat with the other Patients. This could take twenty minutes or two hours. It's a bit of pot luck either way!

My family hired me the TV/Telephone gadget for two weeks at a time. This was great as the Commonwealth Games were taking place in Glasgow and being a sports fanatic, I loved every moment of the coverage. What a great games the England Team had finishing in first place with 58 Gold medals, 59 Silver and 57 Bronze, a Grand total of 174 Medals and a multitude of records, the Aussies were 2nd placed 37 medals behind whilst Scotland managed 4th place with a total of 53 medals of which 19 were Gold.

On my second day in Ward 6, our friends Maureen & George came to see me, alas I was taken ill and started to vomit a little in their presence.

It did not last long but my stomach was upset for the next couple of days. At one point it was thought that I had lactose intolerance. It turned out that I didn't get on too well with the Hospital food, nothing new about that then!

On day 9 in the Royal Hallamshire, the 13th July my niece who is also my god-daughter, Samantha came along with her husband Jonathan, to visit, It was really nice to see them. They brought sweeties……yummy!......a Nice treat!

At this stage I must point out that Maureen was at my side at every visiting opportunity, also regular visitors were Denise & Bill ,Michael & Jon and our Grandchildren Jack, Annabell & William. I had the most fantastic Family Team possible. My brother Alan & wife Pauline were always regular visitors with wonderful Jelly babies or Fruit jellies etc, I was treated like a horizontal lord and believe me, I needed treats. You feel totally *hopeless & helpless*, when in that situation. What with not being able to move the left side of my body at all and not having sufficient core strength either leaves you feeling so dependant on others. Something you need to accept, along with getting your mind mentally re-adjusted to the possible future ahead.

It was about this time that when our Mike and Jon visited that Jon started trying to get my weak leg working a little better. He would lift the leg up, bend the knee and I would power it straight, we did this on most visits for a couple of months. It sure did help build up the Quadriceps around my knee for the strength needed to sit to stand or walk.

On the following day, two more of my relatives Alma & Joseph called. This was a lovely surprise as we only ever see each other at Weddings & Funerals; maybe they thought it a good idea to see me just in case they were on holiday, if I pegged it. Probably not, but best be on the safe side Eh!.

After their visit I was taken for another "Check on the Brain" MRI scan........Yes the walnut was still working!

During the afternoon of the same day, I was taken for the first of my 3 times a week Physiotherapy Sessions. This is not anywhere near the amount needed, but what with cutbacks in the NHS, that is the only amount of time allocated to me. A physio named Jack came along and fed various pieces of the hoist padding around me; they fetched a mobile hoist, attached me to it and lifted me up to place me in a wheelchair for transportation to their Gymnasium.

This hoisting was a regular occurrence, during my stay in hospital, and one that I referred to as my *Air Yards*. Once at the Gym I was hoisted onto a physio's plinth, a table very similar to massage couches. We were joined immediately by the physio's assistant, Vivian. They sat me upright to start to help strengthen my core-stability. "**SIT UP TALL**" is the command, (one that will accompany you through life). This was a case telling me to "Sit up tall" and with Viv behind me, making certain that I did not collapse in any direction, her job was basically to get me to move about and then sit up straight again. It took a couple of weeks to build up my core, strong enough, not to flop about. They worked on it for about 10 minutes on each of my journeys to the Gym.

The first thing you get taught when trying to stand up from a sitting position is for you get your *chest weight over your knees* otherwise the move just does not happen, and at the same time push up with your good arm or two if you have both working. So always get this manoeuvre to the foremost part of your thinking before you even attempt to stand.

After my first core building exercise, I was asked to stand with my back to this plinth; they placed another plinth at a right-angle to this, on my right-hand side. "Now Roger we want you to take a few steps forward" and for a first time it was quite successful. That is I didn't finish up on the floor.

Then I did another 3 steps forward and also 3, sort of backwards, but with a lot of help. After a while they hoisted me back into the wheelchair and returned me back to the Ward. More ***Air Yards***. It was Teatime and I was *"Cream-crackered"*

I must have registered at least 150 of these hoisted ***Air Yards*** by the time that I left Hospital…………but no free trip anywhere apart from Oak Lane Rehabilitation Centre.

Tea was a cross between a Shepherd's Pie, a Fish Pie and something that I could have thrown together! If not Yuk! then it was certainly different. Once Maureen had arrived the meal became just an historical *faux pas*, as we chatted away, absorbed in each others company.

The following morning I got weighed, it scales read 13stones 13 pounds a little less than the 16stones 3 pounds that I carried on the outgoing flight to Turkey. Two reasons for the weight loss, Lack of appetite (you make your own mind up as to why) and the massive amount of muscle loss due to the lack of any form of strength activity.

CHAPTER 5 / Day 22

12th July 2014

Lung Problems

Every time a member of staff came to ask me to turn, an often used practice with long term patients to keep their chests clear and to avoid bed sores, they would say "which is your best way to turn for me" onto my weak left was the way to go. So this is what I did, but on this particular day I was hit with a horrendous pain in my back. I thought that I had pulled a muscle there, what with all the pulling I had to do on the cot sides just to turn over on request. I was totally convinced of this, but the Doctor who came to see me thought differently. An hour later I was taken firstly for Brain scan (found in decent condition!) then for a Lung scan. They injected with a radio-active dye, which gives you a lovely warm feeling and helps to make clear pictures of the Lungs. This fluid disperses naturally and has no side-affects. When the Lung piccies were scrutinized, the Doctor realized that he was right in his suspected diagnosis. Yes I had various sized blood clots on one of my Lungs, good gracious any more good news! The outcome of this diagnosis was that I needed two injections daily of Dalteparin, A morning dose of 10000 units of 3ml of the solution and a further 7500 units in the evening. One to the left-hand side of my body and one to my right-hand side. This would continue for 6 Months. Four months of which I performed myself. I asked if I would need a follow up Lung scan to see whether the injections had worked. "No! no need to follow up the Dalteparin as this will clear the Blood clots up within this 6 months period, for sure! Once the injections commenced, the pain started to subside and was gone completely in 36 hours. That was a pain I would not inflict on my worst enemies, it was excruciating. It pulsated and when the pain struck, I could neither talk nor breathe, you just had to await it abating. A real eye-opener to extreme pain! Ever since the introduction on Day 1and the insertion of the catheter in Turkey to drain away my *liquid waste,* I have not had to concern myself with this routine exercise, as the pipe to the bag was all that was needed. However today the 14th August is **Flip-Flow day**, the day that the staff, a pretty young student nurse, under supervision attached a piece of equipment that allows me to determine when I actually controlled my own urine flow. This entailed a piece of tube with a valve control in the middle of the external sector, which I could open and close, to appease my bladder. It took a couple of days to get used to doing this function for myself, one handed. Generally speaking, it was a lot easier to Pee before this new fitment. However I had to start the long road to normality somewhere! The flip-flow was used for about just under a fortnight. The Catheter, with the flip-flow attachment, was removed by the same young nurse who had fitted it, without any pain or discomfort; this was Day 38, the 28th July. Then I was in total control of this function. It always takes a little longer than you think to empty your bladder, so the tip is always give yourself an **extra minute** when you are using a bottle for this purpose. It's a big responsibility being in charge of your our water works, and it is something that often catches you out! i.e. *Chapped thighs!!*

Last thing at night, staff would ask who wanted a bottle or two for the night ahead. Well, both Gerry and I would use any amount up to 7 or 8 per night, *getting our monies worth out of the NHS.* The least we ever needed was about 4 bottles each. Why when you relieve yourself 2 or 3 times during the day you need so many bottles at night, puzzled us both. One night after use, I picked the used bottle up to put on my table for collection, I got saturated! The bloody thing had a hole in the bottom and it went all over me and the bed. The nursing staff had to change both me and the bedding. Gerry had a very similar incident happen to him. After these incidents we would hold them up to the light and check for holes. Then 3 days later, when half asleep, I pick one up to check for holes but alas it was part used or even part emptied, and I got a face full of the stuff............Error!!

We all thought more care was needed during future inspections!

CHAPTER 6 / Day 42

1st August 2014

The next few weeks passed without too much special or unusual happening. Loads of regular visitors and physiotherapy, alas the physio sessions were only about 3 times each week. This is not enough for patients that have just had their worlds turned upside down, and need all the help available. You need this therapy, EVERYDAY, but with the NHS in financial melt-down, you couldn't get anymore than anyone else. This is poor so was the lack of nursing staff, daily. No one wants to work in the Stroke Wards, they are hard work and very physical, with the lifting and turning of patients, helping them to sit up or turned to get on a bed pan etc, etc. All a bit of a struggle for the staff, especially the ones with bad backs, and most of the nurses appeared to have these.

My new best friends were all doing the very best they could. Gerry had managed about six yards with sticks and a physio behind keeping a close eye on him. Abdul was walking about fairly good at this time and was about to be shipped out the Oak Lane Rehabilitation Centre, the next stop on the road to home. He was replaced in Bed A, by Keith Thomas an octogenarian with lots of problems, not just his stroke but other medical issues. Eddie got to go home 3 days earlier on the 29th July. His replacement was a businessman called, Derek Jackson. Derek was always on the phone doing deals or just talking about them. Interesting! But not always my cup of tea, as no good Stock market tips were ever passed on. After a day or two we realized that Derek's stroke had left him with a few mental as well as physical problems.

Day 43
Saturday 2nd August 2014

A Break through ……………..I was allowed to leave the Ward with the use of a Wheelchair being pushed by Maureen. They allowed us to go downstairs to the cafeteria. I indulged in my first proper cup of **coffee and a biscuit** since that bloody awful day back in June. Gosh my very first trip in a wheelchair and I get goodies as well. **This was truly a Red Letter day for me.**

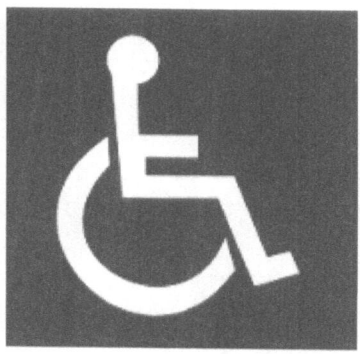

The following day I was in the Wheelchair again, first we went to "D" floor to have a nosey around the staff canteen/dining room……boring! Then down to ground where we went for a little push outside to take in some of the lovely sun. Great! Then into the café once more for coffee etc, after which we ascended back up to SU1. Instead of going straight onto the ward we went for a look around Sheffield from an exalted position in the Day Room, trying to pick out all known areas to the East of the City. It is really a fascinating pastime to actually settle these details firmly in your brain. Then the next time you do this again, you change your mind..........good fun!

"SIT UP TALL"

We continued with the routine, wash/breakfast or breakfast/wash, TV, Gym or not Gym then Mrs.T, then lunch before our daily wheelie trip down to the café and the sunshine. We were usually met or followed down by our other visitor(s) either Alan & Pauline, or Jack, or Annabell or William. This routine carried on until the 10th August, Alan's birthday, the day that Pauline had sprayed her eye with an adhesive substance rather than her contact lens solution, big error as the lens was stuck solid! The reason was that both the bottles were identical in all ways apart from their labels. We met Alan down by the café and followed him the eye department where Pauline had been for quite a while and was being attended to. Fortunately, she was soon sorted out and her eyesight saved, with the usual warning "Don't do that again". Pauline had to wear an eye patch for a couple of days to allow the eye to "Restore" itself. The eye inflammation last about 5 or 6 days then it was back to normal.

About my third week in the Royal Hallamshire I was asked to take part in a new special electrically operated inflatable foot splint. This was to try and get some movement with the foot and to assist in the onward challenge of the dropped foot. I tried this for about 10 days, as this was all the time available for this trial. Alas it did not seem to improve my situation, but others ... Maybe!

Monday brought a new challenge. An occupational Therapist came to ask me a lot of question which I had to answer. A *Compos Mentis* test to check whether I had got my Brain was in gear or not. I answered all questions correctly apart from one when I said that World War II was 1939-1946 and not 1939p- 1945, which I corrected, after a prompt. Then I had to copy a wooden puzzle from associated blocks……..accurately done in a couple of minutes. I said I would bet that most of the staff would have struggled with that one. No comment was forthcoming from the O.T.

I passed with 92/93% the War dates beat me to the 100%.

"SIT UP TALL"

About the time of the evening meal I was told that the following day Tuesday I would be going to Oak Lane Rehab Centre. So they needed to start me using a Rotunda to help with my Transfers. Transfers as in getting from bed to chair or chair to bed or wheelchair to Loo etc.After the meal the Rotunda arrived. The staff helped me to slide off of the bed, and with their help to stand totally upright on the Rotunda and told to hold on tight. The equipment which had a rotatable footplate would be rotated 90 degrees or indeed 180 degrees and locked off. This made the Transfer to a chair, quite easy. However some staff made it harder to hold on to the Rotunda by turning a little faster than was probably, safe to do so.(Not the Hospital staff but others later in my story.) Or were they just checking out my strength, balance or ability to sustain this movement.

Mmm I wonder!

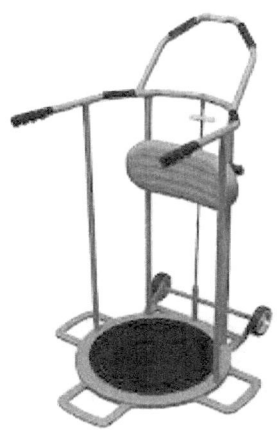

Gosh! What a busy day

Monday was a day of receiving information about Oak Lane and how good it was and what they would do with or for me. Trying to gather all of my gear together, collecting my transfer forms and my list of medications, having a shower, my first for 52 days was a strange treat of sorts and one that would be repeated regularly in the future, and practicing some Rotunda transfers.

CHAPTER 7/ DAY 53.

TUESDAY 12TH AUGUST 2014.

OAK LANE REHABILITATION CENTRE. TRANSFER DAY.

After my Breakfast of Cereal & Toast, I started to mentally prepare myself for today's short but yet very significant journey to the Rehab Centre and the next step in my quest to get home. Lily my favourite nurse arrived, to help in collecting all my stuff together for the move and helping me change into some Street clothes for that move. Lily said that she would be back to wish me Good Luck before I left but she never made it. Lunch came and went and then at 14:30 hours the Ambulance crew arrived to take me to me new home. It was about 15:30ish when we arrived at the Centre which is a large stone built Mansion, originally owed by the then Lord of the Manor, Lord Suffolk, This old City home of his was presented to the NHS 12 years ago, after some personal tragedy.

   I was met on arrival by Nurse Miss Georgina Edwards, a lovely looking young lady with a really good figure, who I later found out to be a Grandmother of three……..Hospitals must play with your conscience and general perceptions of people and life, it certainly did with mine. Confused or What!

   Miss Edwards took me through by wheelchair to my Room No.10, which was situated very near to the nurses' station. This was so they could keep a close eye on me. Soon after my arrival our Alan & Pauline came to assist me settle in and await Maureen's arrival in the early evening. Afterwards the visit they took Maureen home, which was really good of them, as they live 15 miles in the opposite direction from home, across and out of the City. "SIT UP TALL"

I saw Abdul on day 2, but poor old Abdul seemed a lot worse than he did in Hospital, but he had found another Indian Gentleman to chat with. They had curries for their evening meals. Something that I did, once I realized I was allowed to, it was certainly a lot better than the other food available. Abdul's walking seemed to have got worse; this I believe was the lack of assistance/help in this Centre.

Because of the problems associated with transfer arrivals I.E cross-contamination all new patient arrivals had to stop in their own rooms for the first two days. This is not too bad as the room had a small television, did I say small no **Tiny** is what I meant to say, but it was better than nothing, just!

The room had a well equipped bathroom with Toilet, Shower of sorts and a wash basin. Actually the shower was just a hose down area, as the shower head did not work efficiently and therefore removed.

In the room itself, apart from the Hospital bed were 2 comfortable lounge chairs, a wardrobe and a couple of drawers, upon which stood the television. The room also had a foot stool and a table on wheels and a Bathroom transfer chair. This was tubular steel chair on lockable wheels with a padded back and commode seat, which was used to transport me to the Bathroom for the Loo, Sink or Shower, it was very useful indeed. The room faced the rear of the property and over looked an area of grass, the back end of

Suffolk Park and a few private garages, could be worse I suppose.

I must have been a "Good Boy" as they staff allowed me to join the other inmates on the following day for the evening meal. That was good to talk to my "New best friends". One of the first things you notice upon arrival at the "Feeding Station" aka the Dining Room, is that you are just one of many who are all trying to come to terms with having a stroke and realizing that there are lots in the same boat as you.

Some however have multiple problems and not just a one-sided weakness or as I would have called it paralysis. These problems amounted to such as things as speaking difficulties or poor eating/swallowing, or hearing, or vision problems as well.

The Daily lunchtime food was mainly sandwiches of various fillings or Jacket potatoes none of these made much of good impression on me. The Evening meal varied more, but still did not impress me. After my evening meal I was taken straight back to my cell, I mean room! To prepare for the Night ahead, from 6 p.m. it was "Do you want to get in bed yet" NO! I replied "Please come back much later". As I have said before, I was very lucky with visitors,

"STAND TALL!" the new command

Maureen came every afternoon and every evening. A lot of the time I was in there, the local Supertram, stopped nearby, but alas was actually out of commission. The Supertram Company was busy replacing some of the tracks, as they were 20 years old, and getting very worn. So my missus had to walk from the City centre to the Rehabilitation Centre, fortunately the weather was fine and mostly sunny throughout all of my Hospital and Rehabilitation stays.

What a good summer that was!

Either Michael & Jon or Denise & Bill would take it in turns to take Maureen home at the end of the evening visiting time. I had the most fantastic support team behind me, My Wife, Brother, Son, Daughter, Grandchildren and Friends would all visit me regularly. I must have been the only *Guest"* at Oak Lane who had visitors at both Visiting Sessions each and every day that I was in their establishment, I was a rarity that you saw or heard the same visitors on a regular basis.

Friday 15th August, saw my first visit to their Gym. It was a similar size to the Hospitals Gym but had more types and variations of equipment, there were also windows, which they did not have at the Royal Hallamshire. My first session was obviously to test my ability to stand and control my core status. Firstly they got me sat on a plinth with assistant Ruth placed behind me to assist my core, should it be needed. Whilst Joanne Sutton the head physiotherapist, something I found out later, stood in front issuing instructions to Ruth and controlling any and all forward movements, When Joanne was satisfied as to my core strength she asked and indeed tempted me into a standing position, this I did, not too good, but I had and then we tried me walking a few places. Joanne held my hands out front of me and Ruth followed behind with my wheelchair. This was so that I could sit after I had done my requested five paces to rest. Well done Rog!

"STAND TALL!"

I was taken back to Room 10. This all took about 40 minutes in total and a sense of euphoria descended upon me as did a very fulfilling tiredness. I was awoken to the sound of "Roger. Are you coming to the Restaurant for some Lunch" said Hilda one of the staff, "yes of course" was the answer. When we had had our Lunchtime presentation of comestibles, it was back to your cell for the afternoon mix of Antique and or cooking programmes on the telly or reading. This is quite hard during the early period after stroke because of your lack of concentration; it does of coarse improve with time and effort.

Then my loving wife would arrive and bring me up-to-date on any news or local happens or just plain gossip. Then my beautiful granddaughter Annabell arrived straight from work, bringing jelly babies again. And saying things like "don't worry Grandma I will come down everyday to look after Grandad for you, this of course never did happen but it was a wonderful thought! Annabell was working full time so impossible to do, however a lovely thought.

I usually agreed to get in bed about 10p.m, but continue to watch the box until I was sleepy except on Saturdays when I would switch the Telly off after Match of the Day had finished. The night staff would always supply me with a couple of urine bottles for the night. They would come in to see if I was okay or if any bottles needed to be emptied.

The Art of putting me/helping me to get into bed went as follows:

I would be wheel-chaired to the side of the bed, a Rotunda brought for me to stand, whilst standing I would be turned 90 degrees so that I could to sit upon the bed adjacent to my pillows. The Nighttime nursing assistant would lift my legs upon to the bed whilst I lie down, cover me up and and place my table next to me with all the necessary stuff. Such as TV remote control, urine bottles, water and any other items I needed for the night.

During the night staff would have a look in to see if I needed anything or I was okay or empty any used bottles. The process in the morning was bed to Rotunda, **"STAND TALL!"** Rotunda to shower transfer chair, then after the bathroom visit it was shower transfer chair to rotunda, rotunda to wheelchair, wheelchair to brekkie, lovely!

You would be awakened each morning by the noisy arrival of staff at or about 06:30hrs. From about 07:15 after their meeting with & take over from the night staff, they would commence getting people out of bed. This process usually finished in time for all to be taken through to the Dining room for their Breakfasts. However, occasionally it did not go to plan and you could be stuck in your room all morning, with staff going through to the Kitchen, to fetch you some food (i.e. Toast and cereal usually). On these days you probably did not see anyone else until Lunchtime. But you could be lucky if it was your day to have "Physio". Which was very good, the physiotherapy staff really worked hard for you but it was never enough.

IF AFTER YOUR INITIAL RECOVERY FROM A STROKE YOU OUGHT TO RECEIVE DAILY OR EVEN TWICE DAILY PHYSIOTHERAPY then I am sure that all patients would get a better chance of recovery,. This in the long term, I am sure, would save the NHS a massive amount of money, rather than being **"too little too late"**.

"STAND TALL!"

Round about 08:00 hrs on the 19th August staff came to tell me I was going to have to change rooms, Apparently Room 10 had a special bed and that bed was now needed for a patient more urgently needy of it, than me! So after breakfast I would be taken to the Lounge whilst they deep cleaned both Room 10 and my new home, Room 15, The Lounge was a very pleasant room with lots of chairs, a big telly and lots of book shelved full of interesting books.

One was about China which I would have liked to look at, but alas all these comfy chairs and other furniture just blocked the way…………………..No thought had ever gone into this room on behalf of their Inmates/Patients. In fact the room was only used for the purpose that left me stuck there, twiddling my thumbs for a couple of hours before Lunch and a further two, after lunch. No one called in to see me until Maureen arrived mid afternoon. Suddenly the Fire Alarm went off creating it's cacophony of noise, a staff member popped their head around the door, "no need to go anywhere as it's just a practice". Straight afterward this alarming intermission, we were allowed to go to my new cell……….

CHAPTER 8 / Day 60

19th August 2014

Room 15, the furthermost room away from the Nurses Station. I suppose that this is good news in a way, but a lonely place for any patient who got this room, that did not receive regular visitors. The Room with its yellow painted walls and cheap yellow G. plan style curtains. Which looked like they had been bought as a job lot from a Pound store, and crap curtain tracks probably designed by Class 4C or younger? The curtains were always getting pulled off the track, as the stoppers were missing. My visitors were always re-attaching them for me to stop those prying eyes peeping in! The staff were so busy that unless you actually rang for assistance, then they did not have time to even look in on you at anytime during the day. The room itself was pretty much of a muchness, but the new view, was of a courtyard where Matron liked to park her big Posh car, good job Eh! It looked over the entrance, where the evening visitors would try to gain access with the help of a Buzzer This buzzer rang in the Nurses Station/Office as is also where the Weekday 9 - 5 Occupational Therapists Desks happen to be situated. These Therapists had the responsibility to organize your homes both inside and outside, so that you could cope well and be safe, when you were allowed to go home.

    To do this they would visit your home and tell your partner what they were going to do to help you, whether you really wanted these or not. But you would accept their recommendations as they had the knowledge and expertise, or so you thought!

Don't get me wrong most of the additions that were made we have found very useful but others what have not yet used and may never do so.

During my time in Room 15, I always sat, during the hours of daylight, in my wheelchair. This way I could move about around the room and into the bathroom, when required. Or over to the Television, where I got shaved or put my phone on to charge or tidied my hair or just got another top out of the drawer for later use.

It was a marvelous Summer for weather, but did the staff ask their charges if they would like to go out into their lovely gardens to look or get some fresh air or just to do a little sun-bathing. **NO**! It really was a shame that it was just not part of their Portfolio, or so it seemed.

You would think that they would encourage you during your daily plight, to move, do exercises and help and assist patients to go outside, when it was good enough weather to do so, and it was good all the time that I was there…..I am sorry to say that this was not the case at Oak Lane Rehab Centre, none whatsoever. Not one Patient, whilst I was there, was actually taken out into theirs grounds ……………Diabolical!

One day I asked the "Matron" about Wi-Fi, as I and others at the Centre had "Android Tablets" and we would like to use the Internet and send Emails etc…………"You can't have it as our Security is not good enough to stop you looking at our Accounts etc"……….God what a load of Tosh!

So NO lounge or big Telly/NO fresh Air/Sun/Wifi and to top it all the Matron changed the Visiting hours to 18:30 in the evening from 18:00 until 20:00, because the staff eat at this time and altogether, not staggered as is normal in these situations. So she reduced the visiting hours by 30 minutes, if you could get in that is! When visitors arrived they had to wait outside until a member of staff could find time or be bothered to respond to the buzzer.

Just one of the many reasons that it is hard to find anybody, who stayed in this Centre that actually enjoyed their time there! Most just endured it!

However the good news was that with Michaels' help we now had a Stair Lift fitted at home. We had paid a sum of money for its fitting/removal, as and when we had finished with it. We now pay just £40 per Month rental.

It's a good thing that I got some <u>decent</u> Physiotherapy, it helped me a lot both with my thought patterns and my physical strength to be able to stand and walk a little with a physio assistant in front holding my hands out the physiotherapist on a low stool helping to place my feet in correct places. Another exercise was, I would lie on a plinth, and the head physiotherapist would bend my legs up towards my chest, she would then kneel on the Plinth and place my feet on her chest. She would then press her weight down on my legs and I had to support her full upper body weight for about 4/6 minutes. "Don't let me drop", she would say. "I won't" I would say, "as I now where you will land" Mmm Squeaky voice time. It's always good to have a laugh during a hard physio session or indeed any other time as it relaxes you and makes you feel a lot better and it increases and heightens your mood and pleasure.

On about my third trip up to the Gym we started to practice seating transference, this was done using a slide board. These heavy duty plastic boards were about 30 inches long and 15 inches wide. They formed an arc shape and the idea was to put ones good hand onto the board, which they would place as a bridge between two plinths, and shuffle ones bottom along it, hand bottom, hand bottom and again and again until you reached your destination i.e .Plinth No.2. It takes a little time to get your body doing these different manoeuvres, but it is well worth the effort for future activities, and there will be lots of all those.

Occasionally my afternoon visitors, Maureen, Alan, Pauline or my close mate Peter would come up to the Gym to watch and encourage my attempted gymnastics or gymnastisms or whatever it was, that I did. The gym sessions were all gratefully accepted, be they 40 minutes or 90 minutes in duration. Every session was of great benefit for the stroke survivor who wanted to get going as fast as possible and to get home. We all realized that the sooner you could get home the faster would be your recovery. **THERE IS NO PLACE LIKE HOME!** You tend to push yourself for longer spells when at home and become a little more daring, one hoped!

My family would often at weekends push me into the Sunny gardens where I could take in the Air and indeed top up the rather fading tan, from my Turkish Trip.The really fortunate patients, who had been shown how to transfer in and out of cars, got to be taken out by their families for an hour or two on their weekend visits. I had yet to endure a little more time at this Centre!

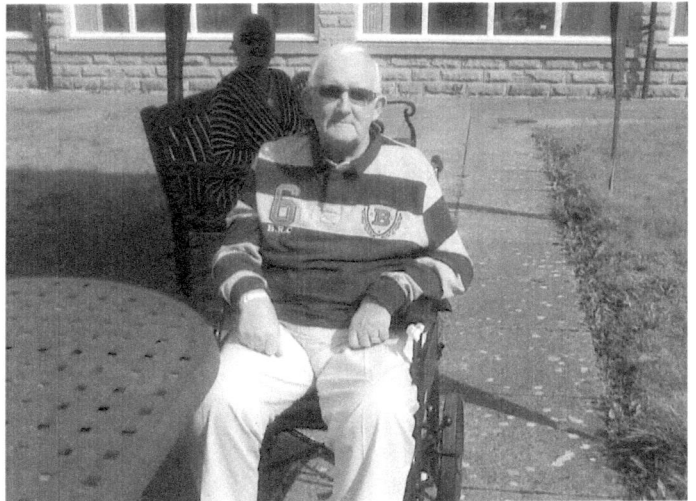

Taking in the Sun, thanks to Alan & Pauline.

On the 25th August my old pal Gerry arrived from the Royal Hallamshire. He was booked to get to the Centre before me but had a couple of health setbacks. Gerry got my old Room no.10. The chap that I had had to move out for had actually had a bit of a relapse and had to go back to Hospital. He later returned and was given the special room No.1.

This room was bigger and lighter than the others and was better equipped to cope with his particular problems. It had its own bed to chair(s) hoist and one of those massage chairs to stop you getting bed sores/ulcers, which happens when we cannot move for ourselves.

I was good to have a catch up with Gerry. He told me about how the others are we left behind in SU1 and of my replacement, a bloke called Dave who had arrived from Chesterfield with not only had a Stroke but broke an arm in the fall. Poor old Lad! Gerry and I always sat at the same table for meals and chat merrily about our Physio Sessions, and all other topical topics on the news or in the press generally. I asked him whether he had made a decision about trying to get back to be able drive at any point.

He said that he and his wife and family all agreed that he should not drive again, safety was foremost in their minds. Just get lifts from the family or Taxis or Community transport or any other form, but definitely not by himself. I said that I would like to be able to hold a Driving License again, one day.

When next I visited Jo the head Physiotherapist, she worked on my arm to try and get a little more response out of it, it was not much better than before but a glimmer of hope raised its head. Then I did the "support your physio" exercise. Good power in the legs generally and certainly getting more in the weaker left one.

Then I tried my standing on my weaker leg whilst trying to kick a ball with the other. To my amazement I sort of did this, without falling over, but there again I had not fallen over yet, and had no intension of starting.

"STAND TALL!"

Saturday the 30th August was, as usual on a Saturday **"BRUNCH DAY"** This meant that we got Bacon sarnies or Sausages if we wanted them. EVERYBODY wanted them, if only for a change from the usual, followed by Tea or Coffee. Both Saturday & Sunday I got to be pushed out in the grounds by either Alan & Pauline or Maureen, struggling with the fact that it was not the easiest of terrains to push a small-wheeled wheelchair, which is the type that I had been allotted.

On Monday 1st September 2014, the Sister in charge came to see me about self medicating, which is keeping control over my own Pills and at the same time. The sister said she needed me to start doing my own twice daily Injections of Dalteparin, 10000 units in the morning and 7500 units in the evening. This is a daunting task at first but you soon get used to the routine, but the bruises that they create do last a long time.

Not much happened during the next couple of weeks. Three meals a day, Physio three times a week, put curtain back on track three times a day (probably), taken outside in the sun three times a week, Loo three times day, Shower aka a Hose down a couple of times a week.

My Doctor called every Wednesday to reassess all of his Patients and make whatever decisions were deemed necessary. Things carried on like this until the 3rd September (Day 75) when after requesting to go home for the last three weeks I was told that the Doctor agreed that if the Occupational Therapists could arrange my home care package, I could go home the following week. However, they could not get it sorted out in time with the home care team until the following week. Before being allowed to go home/ dispatched/aquitted/released/freed, one or two things happened. Firstly the Physio's got me practicing my walking, with one of them holding my arms in front of me and Jo was watching where I was placing my feet. I managed about 18 yards on about three occasions, one of which was by me and one of these strong ladies holding my left arm whilst I was given a Quad stick to aid my stability, in my right hand. Earlier in the Gym.I had I also practiced standing and looking at 90 degrees, this was to see if I could hold my balance whilst turning which destabilized me, we did a lot of this turning to look at the back wall or at a light fitment or towards a window or rolling a ball on a plinth with it under my one handed control. We had done a few of these exercises over the past three weeks, but it became more intensive when it became agreed to allow me to go home.

On Friday the 12th the one and only male Physiotherapist there, whom I never got to exercise me, asked if I would like to have a go at a Wii that he was setting up in the Lounge for after lunch. I agreed anything for a change and it would be interesting to see if I could do anything at all on this Wii. So with Gavin the physio helping me stand on the Wii board and locking my left hand on a zimmer frame, I did the same on the other side with my right hand. The game that we played was about penguins flipping out of the sea onto moving Ice floes. Your job was to wobble these icefloes by weight transference on the Wii board to keep the Penguins on these floes and not let them slide off. Awkward to do, but fun also........I had about a dozen or so goes and finished as the highest scorer of the day, just beating Gerry. <u>Smashing!</u>

The following Wednesday four of us were asked if we fancied a game of Dominoes by Ruth the junior Physiotherapist. So Gerry, Gordon, Aidan and me went through to the overflow Dining Room where Ruth was awaiting us with the Dominoes. Gordon sat with Gerry and me most meal times Aidan did occasionally. Gordon a lovely fellow who went into the Royal Hallamshire for a fairly routine operation and finished up having a stroke which did not affect his body and limb movement massively but it did leave him, not able to talk in any form of coherent way. What a damned shame as Gordon was really talkative but we could not understand a word, really frustrating for him. Although his wife could understand what he wanted, when she was there, of coarse. I digress; we played basic dominoes for about an hour and was most enjoyable. Aidan who we found out had a problem with Dominoes, as in he would select the right domino. For instance if he needed a six he would select a six but place the other end of it against the six! No the other way around Aidan……..he would then wonder way he had put it the wrong way round, he was like that at every go. Gerry or Gordon nearly always won, I am rubbish at Dominoes.

Emotions & Feelings so far

Part 1. Chapters 1 - 8

From the first day of my Stroke, to my last day of sleeping away from home, it was like living in someone else's world, not the world that I knew up until that point in my life. The first stages of a stroke are all consuming all rolled into one, you are not well, you do not know what will happen to you. Will you die or maybe worse still, you will turn into a cabbage and become 100% dependant on your wife and the health services. You just lie in bed and during the hours that you feel awake, and I was awake most of the time that I was in the Turkish hospital, but not awake, if you knew what I mean……..just in limbo! When we flew home it was on a Holiday flight, full of tourists who all wondered what was up with the guy at the back of the plane on a stretcher. These tourists would have a lingering look at me on their way to the rear Lavatory and then again on their way back to the safety of their own seats. I was wonderfully manhandled off the plane and back on another plane at Istanbul Airport, but it was very labour intensive. However it was a lot easier at Manchester Airport, primarily because the men there were a lot stronger and I was lifted high, whilst on my stretcher and they somehow got me off the plane without any problems, I still have no idea how they got me around a 90 degree corner to the exit door, but they did. I was not worried in the slightest all the way back to blighty as I knew where I was heading for. Also I had the utmost faith in Dr. Gavin and his organization. The big problem getting from Manchester to Sheffield's Royal Hallamshire Hospital was the knowledge that because of the Tour of France road race taking place from Leeds to Sheffield on that day, that there would be holdups. There were lots of these and the poor Mancunian driver of the Ambulance did not know his way very well and was constantly on the phone to his boss asking for routing help, we got there eventually, thank goodness! At this point along my Journey I had not become weepy at all but I knew that this would alter directly after had gone past a "Trigger Point". But what would that trigger point be, I wondered. ***Some of the time it was just like Brain Freeze but without the Ice Cream.***

PART 2

CHAPTER 9 / Day 90

Thursday 18th September 2014

GOING HOME DAY

After breakfast I went back to Room 15 to gather the rest of my gear together for my Departure for Home. Maureen had been up, as always, the night before, he came with Denise and we decided, what I should wear for my journey today. They took all the rest of my clothes with them and left a holdall for me or a member of staff to pack all the other stuff, which belonged to me. I sat watching the TV for a while. I was then taken for Lunch and told that the Ambulance would collect me about 2:30p.m. so I said goodbye to my fellow diners and Domino players, Gerry whom I had spent many weeks with, Gordon and Aidan.

Then back to my Room to wait, a few members of care staff popped in to say goodbye and Good Luck, as did the Physio staff, I even got a little peck on the cheek from Jo, I was pleased about that as she had given me lots of hope for the future.

The Ambulance arrived more or less on time and off we went to Home, a place that I had not seen for 15 weeks and a place I wondered, would I ever see again!

Upon arrival at home, the Ambulance pulled up outside, Maureen came out to meet and welcome me,

I think that we both had a tear in our eye, tears or joy obviously for my safe arrival home back from the jaws of death/permanent paralysis.

They took me off of the back of the Ambulance in one of their wheelchairs, the one that had been ordered for me was not arriving until later the same afternoon. Then up the two, front pathway, steps and around the side of the house to the back door, which is the most convenient entrance into our home.

They helped me get into a Riser/Recline chair, which was on loan from a lady who worked along side Denise and who we considered along with her husband, good friends.

The very first thing that you notice is how nice home is and how big the TV is. Then we have a nice cup of Coffee, it tastes so good after the liquid cardboard that I have endured recently.!

Maureen tells me about all the alterations that the O.T. from Oak Lane, had set up. A Grip bar and a grab rail in the downstairs toilet, 2 more at the top of the stairs, adjacent to the top of the Stair lift. Two more Grip bars next to the back door on the outside. We have a Hospital bed, set up in our Lounge; fortunately we had room for such, a Commode, a Rotunda and a toilet riser for when I could actually get in there. I was also equipped with a large Quadstick as my walking aid, for when I got good enough walking to be able to use one of these. Later that afternoon, my brand new wheelchair arrived, sent by Taxi. My appointed Home Physiotherapist Lauren turned up to tell me when she would be calling to start my 13 Weeks of her assistance. Oh Goodie! Her first physio session would commence Monday 22nd Sept. 4 days hence.

However at 16: 10 the first of my, 4 times day, Rehabilitation Assistants turned up to see if I needed any help at that time, which I did not. They would call again later to help me to bed or commode or just get ready for bed. When they did call back we had family with us, so yet again no assistance was needed. The following morning they turned up a little later than we thought they would. 09:20hrs. Maureen had already helped out of bed and rotunded me to use the commode, then onto my wheelchair, washed & dressed me and wheeled me to the breakfast table.

The 2 Ladies who called assisted me with my shoes and socks, we had a little chat and then left. Two other RA's (Rehab. Assistants) called at Lunchtime but Alan & Pauline had called to see the set-up and see if we needed anything getting in, Maureen had already organized all of that stuff as well! I was just doing a few of my Rotunda Squats, when they arrived, so they saw that I was well and active. The night time helpers came at 19:30hrs, they were not needed at that time, we would attend to my getting into bed.

This was what happened on many days, but on other occasions they would attend to me. The first of the four daily calls was to assist me wash and dress. I would be helped from bed on to the Rotunda, then in to my wheelchair to the commode. After which it was back on to the Rotunda. This time it was a case of stripping me naked and washing me all over whilst I held on to the said Rotunda, drying me off then I sat down on my wheelchair, which was directly behind me, whilst I was dressed, then taken to the table for Breakfast The second call was to see if I needed the commode again or if they needed to get any lunch ready. Maureen always produced this, but the visit did give me a time to Build up my Quads a bit more by doing squats whilst I yet again stood up to and held on to the Rotunda. You have to hold on tightly to this piece of equipment just incase it hadn't been locked off fully because if it hadn't been it could turn a little and you could finish up in an **"ACE OVER BASE"** just like being thrown off the waltzer and landing flat on your back.

The Third call was at Teatime and this was the same carry on as Lunchtime. The Fourth was to assist me get into and attain a comfortable position in the Hospital Lounge bed.

Come Monday Lauren arrived promptly at 11:10a.m, just a slight delay because of heavy traffic in the area. She arrived with an assistant named Tina who was a robust Lady and nothing like her name suggests. Lauren on the other hand was a slight built girl in her late twenties who had a couple of children. The elder one was in the Infants school whilst the younger one was in a Nursery Day Care Centre.

Lauren started by getting me to stand by the side of my bed, attached her self to my body, just like a footballing full back would do to a striker, then ask me to take a few paces. I could not move, she had got me locked in! I asked Lauren to unclasp me so that I could move, which she did a little, then I managed to perform the required manoeuvres. We tried this a few times with Lauren detached, she relaxed a little when she could see that I wasn't going to collapse on the floor and generate a whole lot of paperwork for her to do later.

Tina's turn next. Up onto the bed I went to practice my bottom raises. That is, I with Tina's help would lie flat with my knees bent up with my feet placed on the bed, quite near to my bottom.

I had to raise this bottom of mine off of the bed as high as possible, by pressing my feet into the bed and arching my back, then hold for as long as possible. Something like 10 seconds would suffice then back down onto the bed we did this a few more times, before I was too tired to carry on.

This team was to be my regular Physiotherapy support for a full twelve or thirteen weeks period. Lauren was in my opinion too small to be in full control of a not too skinny a man like me, maybe a thinner man or woman but she did not appear to have a lot of confidence in her own ability to give me the necessary confidence with her, if you know what I mean. However with Tina's help, who was of good size, they could just about sort me out between them.

Day 94

This same team came back the following day just after Lunch at about 13:15hrs. Tina did her stuff with me first, she added an extra exercise, that of lifting the bottom up and off of the bed, and then moving it about from side to side. Then I sit up tall on the bed legs dangling down by the side and slide to a standing position on the Rotunda, I then turned 90 degrees so that I could be positioned to sit in my wheelchair. Lauren then wheeled me into the Kitchen for some standing practice. I did this at the far end on the Kitchen, over looking my back garden. I was helped up out of the wheelchair to stand at the worktop. I had to practice swaying from side to side.

This was to try and get the receptors in the sides of the feet to feel this action and send good signals back to the brain about these movements. Hopefully, the brain would start to create new information channels to replace the ones that died during my Stroke.

On the Wednesday, as of last Saturday & Sunday, Family came visiting, as did my old Mate Peter. It's always good to see him, as he cheers me up and makes me feel quite normal, which is an extremely good bonus, especially when you don't feel particularly normal. Peter usually calls after a game of Golf, not that he is any good at it, but he tries hard and more to the point, he enjoys the walk!

Annabell came about 15:30 after she had finished work and brought me some choccies, Gosh! I must have looked too thin.

Friday 26th September saw just Lauren come to administer a little on my rather stiff and extremely toned upper arm and shoulder, she worked hard but it did not seem to reduce any of the toning and was just about the same when she left, I'll see you on Wednesday along with Tina at about 11am.

Family visited at the weekend. Alan & Pauline, also Denise with our Jack, Bill had got a County match, Bill played for the South Yorkshire Veteran Men's Table Tennis Team and has done so for many years.

Jack also plays for the County, but for the Senior Men's Team, but had no matches this weekend. Alan & Pauline called to see how I was progressing and bring Maureen some flowers and Jelly babies for me.

They could see that I was starting to look and feel a lot better, on this my 100th day of the Stroke. All my movement at home was done by Rotunda to Chair or Chair to either Commode or Bed. I could not wait to be able to get to the Loo with its seat riser fitted or not, just to get a little bit of privacy back into my world, but that would have to wait, a little while yet!

The bed was a fully automatically controlled bed, so therefore I could adjust my sleeping position to suit me best. As with all this type of bed the Mattress was fluid resistant and made you perspire a lot, you would wake in the night to urinate and you would be soaked in sweat, every single night that I was in this bed, did I sweat!

Lauren & Tina came on Wednesday and we practiced transfers from bed to wheelchair and then to commode a few times then it was onto the bed for Tina's specialty, the bottom lifts and we actually tried a new type of exercise. This was on where I lie on my side, knees together and then I had to separate my knees and hold a gap for just about 5 seconds at first but this would get extended in time to about 30 seconds. This got you breathing heavily and created a bead of sweat on the brow, tiredness prevailed after a full hour with these Ladies doing there best. Tina came back on the Friday and we did her routines once more, but slightly better than previous.

Every weekend and indeed many days during each week, we had visitors to see us both and talk about how the week had gone and what exercises I was or had been doing with them and without them. I tried working my arm/fingers a lot of the time and with a modicum of success, plus my 3 or 4 daily squat sessions on the Rotunda. These help a lot with the leg strength that is needed many times each day.

When I came out of the Rehab.Centre we were told not to do any improvements at home until "Stay Put" had been to see what we would need to assist me getting out and about, <u>so we didn't do anything, we waited!</u>

Lauren & Tina came on Tuesday the 7th October and lo & behold something a little different, mind you at our request. Tina pushed me to the bottom of our stairs and with her help and of coarse the quadstick, managed to position myself on the Stair lift seat, "Well Done Rog." Then back onto the wheelchair and I was taken to the Downstairs Toilet. This Toilet was only established earlier in the year, because we needed one to stop both us and anybody else, having to traipse through the lounge to get to the bathroom upstairs.

The toilet was originally our Pantry and about a 2 foot length off of the Kitchen. Jon came up with the idea as he was until recently, an Interior Designer. We thought the space available for this job would never be sufficient, but it was, and we are most grateful for his expertise. So Tina, with great difficulty managed to get me into this space, in the wheelchair. I stood holding the grab rail and then with a slight turn to the left I could hold the grip bar with my right hand. I could then attempt to stand and wee. I different task but it was quite successful considering the spectators viewing the event. My first urination stood up, but with help!

Wednesday came and another visitor was due. This was the Social Services to set up the onwards Care Package to carry on from the Stroke Team when they finished their time with me. We set their Daily Visits to 2 with just the Lunchtime and the Late evening calls. Maureen could manage to get me up & washed and transported to the commode or my Lounge chair or the Dining Table and also to Rotunda me back to bed at night. I was still using a bottle into which I would urinate whilst sitting in or standing up from my chair, for a little while longer yet!

CHAPTER 10/ Day 110

THURSDAY 9ᵀᴴ OCTOBER 2014

The day after saw the Physio girls do the same transfers as Tuesday and also transferred me to my Lounge Chair. Later in the afternoon Ruben Steele a top notch O.T. with literally bags of experience and knowledge came on his first trip to see me.

Ruben did some really great work on my Hand/Arm and Shoulder, these felt far more relaxed and even a little useful after he had competed his Session on me. Ruben said that he was surprised that "Stay Put" with the Council help Package, had not yet been in touch and said that he would be in ring them we he got back in the Office. He was also going to check on whether I could have better quality wheelchair or even a self-controlled Power Chair. The answers when they arrived turned out to be NO. By being a one handed patient I could only have an attendant controlled wheelchair and No Power Chair, because I had managed, with my quadstick, to walk the required 10 feet. "The Gods were against me again"!

When Friday 10th October arrived it was just Tina to do some bed work, bottom raises etc .with me, it lasted a mere 25/30 minutes. Also doing the same transfers as Tuesday and also transferred to my Chair.

However the next day, Saturday saw Lauren arrive with a face I had not seen before, Anne. They arrived about 11:00 hrs and I was to practice some more Stepping and Step around transfers, twenty minutes later after many successful attempts. We transferred into the Kitchen and the back window where I was to try one legged stances, with the aid of my trusty quadstik, right leg, no problem, left leg awkward and almost impossible with the dead weight of my left arm, dangling by my side.

A weight of approximately ten kilo's just hanging loose and which needed to be offset by my stance, i.e. a slight pull to the right, to help balance me. Lauren did not like this but it was the only way that I could see to keep me semi-upright. I tried standing perfectly upright but the weight of the arm was just too much. We gave 2 weeks to Care Watch that we would not require their Services any longer.

In the afternoon Michael & Jon came and they helped me to get up stairs, **my first stair lift experience,** and into my Computer room aka The Tardis, "Tardis" because of all the stuff I had there, in this my Control room. I could see the Park that we overlook, a mere 20 yards away. *One hundred and twenty five days since I could last look out onto this sight.* "What a wonderful vista it was" WOW!!

I was then taken by the M & J for a push around the Park, what a fantastic trip, just to visit and view the Park that was so close but yet a million light years away..........................Great!

The problem with getting off our property relied totally on the strength of these men as they had to carry me in the wheelchair around a winding and very awkward pathway, which was also narrow and had sideway restrictions and dodgy footwork positioning as well. "Thanks guys".

The excitement of the Park Trip worked as my hand started to "Grip and Let go" later in the day on Sunday. Monday, Tuesday & Wednesday was just bed to commode to chair transfers with the Lauren &

Tina. Thursday the 16th Oct. was good day. Ruben came with Lauren they worked on my Shoulder and we did transfers from wheelchair to Stairlift.

I even got to go upstairs and with the aid of my Commode/transfer chair actually got on and off of the Family bed. Wonderful stuff.......thanks Ruben!

We went back downstairs and Ruben worked on freeing off my Left Shoulder blade. This had become sort of welded shut due to lack of arm movement and the Subluxation that had occurred with it. Shoulder subluxation is a common occurrence after stroke and can be due to muscle wastage or weakness or spasticity.

Ruben came back alone Friday morning and helped me to walk to the Stairlift then up into the bathroom back to the lift back down and from there to my lounge bed...............What a trip!..........Well done Rog.

In the afternoon Lauren called. She pushed me into the Kitchen to the usual place, placed a thick "Delia Smith" cookbook on the floor in front of me. This book was both large enough and had good thickness for me to practice stepping onto and off again. This was a new thing for me to do! After a few goes she asked me to keep standing on the book whilst I tried some little sideways movements. Not too good at these but will improve with time and plenty of hard work.

Saturday 18th October 2014 Day 119 Since I went on Holiday and 120th Day of my Stroke.

What a wonderful day we had with our Visitors, Denise with both Michael & Jon and later helped me get in the downstairs Loo for the first time. When Alan & Pauline called, it was quite a sunny day so we grabbed our last few hours of the "Light Nights" Sun, just in case we failed to get out again before we changed the clocks to their winter setting.

Monday brought me Lauren & Tina I did a lot of bottom raises and knee raises aka "Clams" as Tina called them. Then to the Kitchen for more stepping up and left leg action, i.e. side stepping.

Tuesday a.m. same as Monday then at 14:30hrs Ruben arrived to work on my Arm/Hand/Shoulder.

Wednesday and only Tina and her Bed work and a little Block stepping, she was now permitted to help me in an upright position as well as flat out on the bed, All on her own, about time too!

On Thursday 23rd October. L & T came in the morning and I proved to them that we, that is Maureen & me could get to the lift, get on and off of the bed and get in and out of the shower without extra help.

This we did slowly but without any problems. Lauren said that I could sleep in the Matrimonial bed tonight, but no "*HANKY PANKY*", no chance I could not move that well or with any sort of Rhythm. Mmmm makes you wish a little though.

Friday saw the start of our "City Wide Alarm" installation, this comprises of a control monitor, which is plugged into the phone lines and a personal wrist alarm call button. If you fall or have any sort of difficult situation, push the call button and their response from their Control HQ is within seconds, asking what problems you have and if they have to come to you, it is usually within 30/40 minutes. Pretty good as the responders could be anywhere within the City. Saturday was the day we finalized our Care Watch Package Team.

On Tuesday "Stay Put", the Council department that was going to help with our outside pathways etc) was due to arrive, but failed to materialize!

Tina came later and we did a few bed exercises, raises & clams mainly, and some more stepping, boring!

Care Watch sent their Assessment Lady, Amanda, on the 28th to fully check me and the house out...........Passed! Their first regular call would commence on the 31st (1 carer twice per day) After she left both auren & Ruben arrived to do a little arm work, then I with their help tried stepping outside my back door. I did this very awkwardly a few times, but it was my *First* go and it was a reasonable go! The Physio. Ladies came and we had a little more of the bed plus step around transfers.

Thursday. 30th October Stroke Day plus 131

The Ambulance arrived at 08:30hrs to take me to the Royal Hallamshire Hospital for my 16 Week? Review, just a bit of a look at me and not a lot other than that. I supposed everything was quite normal as the result was, we will see you again in another 6 months. We then had to wait 3.5hrs for the returning Ambulance, it was rather boring, but we had no option as I needed their help to get into our home once we got there, so a Taxi was just not on at this stage in my recovery.

Friday saw L & T at 10a.m. to do a little more stepping up and down on Delia's Cook book, I am definitely getting better at this. Laureen took me out to her car where I did my first and only official NHS car transfer. It went better than either of us thought it would be. Confidence now abounds!

Care Watch's first call was this Lunchtime and with a further one later would be the last we saw of them until Monday. (1 person Twice daily, Mon.-Fri.)

Not much happened on Saturday but Sunday was a Red Letter day. Michael & Jonathan took us for out for Lunch. I was wheeled to the car and with the car door being opened, I stood up and managed to turn with my back to the front passenger seat, bent in the middle and aimed by bum at the seat whilst keeping my head down. The lads them assisted my stroke leg in as I could manage the other one by myself. All good no problems, this maneuvering was reversed upon arrival at the Parkhead Tavern to enable me in to the Wheelchair for entrance to the Pub Dining Room. We all ate at the Carvery and I really enjoyed this as it was my first Lunch Date, since the stroke, and the food was spot on.

Tina and the infamous Bed workouts on Monday morning followed in the afternoon by Phil a contactor that contactor our Michael had told us about. Phil came to look at what our options would be in laying a pathway across our Garden, which would assist me in my quest to be able to escape our property by Wheelchair. Phil looked at the possibilities and suggested to we could have a concrete path laid from our back gates to out back door. All we have to do is have the Privet Hedge removed and cut a channel across the garden, drop the concrete in this channel and Hey Presto! Phil said that he would sort the Quote out and get back to us in a few days time.

Phil came to look at what our options would be in laying a pathway across our Garden, which would assist me in my quest to be able to escape our property by Wheelchair. Phil looked at the possibilities and suggested to we could have a concrete path laid from our back gates to out back door. All we have to do is Remove the Privet hedge and cut a channel across the garden, drop the concrete in this channel and Hey Presto! Phil said that he would sort the Quote out and get back to us in a few days time.

Tuesday 4th Nov. Both the P. Ladies arrived and helped with my stepping out & back in, my back door. I then did some singles leg raises and some Lounge walks for good measure.

3p.m. and "Stay put" arrived to tell us what they could do. She suggested a Warehouse style Iron gantry to use as a Path, but seeing as the Council had no money left in the pot, one of those would cost us about £2500. Thanks but no thanks! We had waited all this time only to find out what the Council could help with and this was the answer, did not please us, one iota.

5th November was another *first* for me After I had woke up and drank the cup of tea that awaited me. I tackled the start journey for the *first* time. That is, walk into the bathroom and to the Loo and then onto a stool at the sink to get washed, brush my hair, clean my teeth and deodorize. I then walked through to my "Tardis" to answer or eliminate my awaiting *Emails*, before going downstairs for breakfast. This is something that I do most mornings.

Thursday 6th Day Stroke Day plus 138

Tina came to exercise me with doing another million squats and one-leg stands …. Lucky ol' me.

Phoned Care Watch (Amanda) To cease the night calls as these really were now surplus to requirements. Friday was Lauren & Ruben, walking, arm massage and assisting fingers to work a little but not very much.

My very big problem is that whenever I attempt to move my arm/fingers in any way, they just go tense. Later I find out that this tension is called *Toning and will follow me on my journey!*

Friday and Phil rang me with the quote for the New Path, which he said he could do in about a fortnight. We mentioned the cost to M & J, they agreed with us that it was a goer, at that price so we gave Phil to go ahead.

On the Sunday I practiced indoor/outdoor stepping and walking etc. I also tried wiping a few of the dishes, plates etc…….. *A first!*

All the usual routines on Monday with Tina. Ruben called in on the Tuesday to work on my Arm/hand once more plus a bit more stepping up & down off of Delia.

Later that day the services people came to collect my Hospital Bed, Commode, Rotunda and all other attendant bits, no further use needed for these two items! That Rotunda was the bane of my wife's life. It was just so heavy for her to move around the house. I do not know how she coped with it, as it really wore her out mentally and physically. She was glad to see the back of it forever!

Ruben called again on Wednesday, and carried on where he had left off on Tuesday. The following day Lauren called to do some Calf and Achilles stretches and lounge walking. More leg work, balancing & squats on Friday by Lauren.

The following Mon/Tues we did the same again. Later Ruben called with a new shower stool so we went upstairs to try it out. Spot on Ruben, that will be grand.

Thursday 20th November and Phil started our New Path preparations. Concrete poured on Friday. On the Sunday I phoned Care Watch and gave them 2 weeks notice to stop visiting. Not needed any more! Phil was back on the Monday to remove all the wooden edge supports and lay a row of bricks along the lower draft edge of the path to guide the rainwater away onto my lawn and away to soak. Good job done!

In the P.M. Specsavers home service man arrived to test my eyes, this was done and I ordered 3 new pairs, one pair Readers, two pair distance one of which was to be photochromic (i.e. went dark in the Sun).

Lauren & Tina came on Tuesday 25th I told Lauren that we had been out for a meal about 3 weeks ago, It was decided that they wanted another look at my car transfers, this ticks yet another box for them! As a bonus for me they took me for a push around the Park............... Yippee.

The first time since I got home I saw a G.P from my local practice. She only called because I requested a 'Flu Jab at home because I could not get to the Surgery as it is set on a hill and is still too awkward to access.

CHAPTER 11 / Day 159

Wednesday. November 26th 2014

My wife's birthday today, I had a card for her but nothing else at this moment. Care Watch's Mrs. Sample phoned to say that if we wanted today could be the last day that they would call, we accepted that. So no more Care Watch from that moment on. Good, we are now on our own! At around 15:45, with Maureen's help I managed to get into the Kitchen Loo and relieve myself standing upright Alone. Another First! Bunting was put out, cheers went up from the world.

Yippee another wonderful event had happened, well I thought so!

Phil got in touch and recommended a guy to Quote for some railings outside of my back door bordering the concrete path. The Gateman called to see the job in question and said it would only be a couple of days to make what we had asked for and gave us a very good Quote. Which we accepted.

Thursday and Friday Tina came doing some weight transference squats for 20mins a time. Lauren & Ruben came later on Friday and watched me climb in and out of the shower. Another box ticked! For them and for me.

I had previously discussed the possibility of me returning back to driving and he said that he would sort an assessment out for me, Good ol' Ruben.

Also on Friday the gateman came back and fitted the railings, as ordered. Really good service and they were just what we asked for. With an excellent finish to the design and paintwork.

Saturday 29th November more step work with Lauren in Kitchen and she told me that this next week would be the next last week of back-up NHS physiotherapy.

That evening I turned onto my side in bed, just for half an hour, but it was my First time since 20th June, the day before Stroke Day, 162 days in total.

John the Gateman called back as requested on the Sunday as we needed to buy some tall wooded gates. He took the measurements and we agreed on the appearance that we liked, he said "I'll get back with your quote tomorrow" John kept his word and rang with the prices on the Monday. We discussed these with family and agreed to order them. That is, 6ft tall double driveway gates with side pieces to keep the nosey parkers out, a 6ft high "side pathway" gate with 3ft x 2ft panel on the wall at the side thereof.

With the impending situation of no Physiotherapy, I searched the "Net" as did our Denise. We both came up with an Emma Richards as being possibly the best, in our opinion, I also added Gerry Scott to my possible's.

I tried ringing Emma but had no joy so I rang Gerry and she said that she could not help but would talk to Emma for me on Tuesday. Sure enough on Tuesday, I received a phone call from Emma saying that she could call at 11am to assess me as a possible client. Emma came as promised, saw my situation and began to work first on my left hand and then my left foot, then she had me stood up and wanted to see me walk a little… She agreed to accept me as her client. She also apologized for not being available the day before as she was working in Cairo, Egypt. Tina popped in to do a little more work on me, she was surprised to see that I had already hired a private Physiotherapist to continue with my onwards development.

John the Gardner called as requested to give us a price for getting rid of some Ivy that was attached to our driveway stoop and needed to be removed so that the new gates could be fitted, as and when the other John could do them. We agreed a price and his number 2 Billy would call back later that day, to remove the said Ivy.

Tina called in on Thursday and I did squats, walking transfers and some one leg stands in the kitchen at one of the worktops. Lauren and Ruben came on Friday 5th December to help me perfect my shower transfers, which I did 4 or 5 times, getting there! Then they gave me some more massage on the left arm, it works at the time but it does not appear to sustain itself, as the arm's toning is still very much evident.

Sunday 7th December Stroke Day plus 170
HALLELUJAH!

<u>*My First Shower*</u> (I had had showers in Hospital & the Rehab Centre but always with staff, assisting) I did not have any problems getting in or out and sitting on the shower stool, that we had purchased for this purpose. My wife helped me to dry me off, we also dried the floor as I did not need to slip now that I had made it this far.

MONDAY, Tina and Lauren called in to do some more arm work. Tina brought with her a tall walking stick as asked for by Emma; the taller the better, that way you use it as a walking aid and not something to lean upon. Lauren phoned ARC whilst she was with me. ARC is the Assessment and Rehab Centre that is based at the old Nether Edge Hospital, not to be confused with the Royal Hallamshire Hospital where I had stayed. It was the next step towards my recovery and was told that "This was THE place to go".

This once a week visit was on a Tuesday, I would be collected and returned home via an Ambulance. The first time that I would be going was to be the 16th December 2014 and this was to be a morning and afternoon session as it would be for Assessment.

In the afternoon I phoned both Westfield Health to get the go ahead for Emma Richards to administer Physiotherapy (i.e. was she on their list of approved Physio's) she was, so there would be no problems in reclaiming some of my outlay back from my Annual allowance. I then phoned the GP's Surgery to tell then to put on my Records that I would be paying for Physiotherapy and that they would need to complete a form being sent from Westfield and then return as requested, duly signed!

Tuesday 9th Tina came and did a little arm work, then we had the Specsavers guy arrive with my new spectacles. They seemed fine so off he went transaction complete, or so we thought!

Wednesday was the my last day for the Stroke Team, my only visitor was Ruben who came to have yet another go at straightening and relaxing my arm and its Toning, This work on my arm never keeps it relaxed or Tone free for very long. What a damned shame!.

Care Watch notice, finished for good, no more chargeable visits.

I took my 2nd Shower, yippee!

CHAPTER 12 /Day 174

THURSDAY. December 11th 2014

Emma came on Thursday and was straight into my arm then leg then more walking. This Lady is so professional and instills a massive amount of confidence in you. She told me about the potential I had with the little movements that I was actually able to do. From her very first appearance on our threshold, you just believe that you chose the best possible available person for the job.

Gateman came and attached the New gates that he had made. The sort of Walnut finish on them really looked so good. We asked about the side panel for over our side wall which we thought had been ordered. Was as yet not ready as he wasn't sure that we needed them, yes of course we need them John. He apologized for the mess up and said that it could take 8/9 days to complete and fit, we left it with him to do his best.

Ever since I got home from Oak Lane we have been saying that we must get a new Rise/Recline chair for me, if only to let our friend have to loan chair returned to them. Maureen also wanted a Settee that had a foot-up feature for her own comfort. So the decision was made to buy a completely new 3 piece suite. This rankled with me as we had a lovely Dark green leather and wood 3 piece. On Saturday the 13th December Bill & Denise called to take us by car to a specialist furniture shop, to look at the Suites available. I checked them out i.e. sitting in them and getting back out of them, checking their widths and depths and styles, patterns, colours etc. We went home with loads of Pattern Books to make our decision After studying these we made our decision.

The day after Phil came to see us, we paid him for all the outside work that he had organized/completed. i.e. The Pathway and the Gates etc.

This was my first time visit to the Assessment and Rehabilitation Centre (ARC). Today was just about assessing my current abilities so that they could produce a helpful recovery programme. First I was taken in a room for discussions and fill out some paperwork with Jane, one of the Occupational Therapists. Then Maureen and I were told to have a seat in the Lounge/waiting area until I could be seen by a Physiotherapist. We were given a little lunch and set watching to television for an hour or so. Alan the allocated Physiotherapist came to take me/us through to the Gym. This again was to assess my abilities for our once weekly visits. We were then taken home by Ambulance as we had been taken there in the morning we got home at about 16:30hrs. An interesting day, I agreed to go every Tuesday starting the week after on the 23rd Dec. 2014 and would be sooner or later would be seeing an O.T. but definitely be seeing Alan every visit, that's good then. Alan seemed a lot more capable than the Lady who had visited me to administer physiotherapy at home, I shall look forward to that.

The following day was my 68th Birthday; I had lot of phone calls from our extremely loving and busy family but alas only Grandson Jack could call today! Good job really as I was quite tired after for long session at ARC the day before.

Nether Edge Hospital started out in 1844 as a Workhouse to hold 500 inmates. The workhouse later became an institution and then after 1929 was renamed Nether Edge Hospital and as well as having general wards it also had T.B. wards this Sanitoria and later specialized as a Maternity Hospital. Thank goodness that they had up graded the place since those days.

On the 18th my wife went to join her friends at a local Hostelry for a Christmas Lunch. I sat at home watching the Gogglebox for a while and then I had a really nice visit from my God daughters husband Jonathan. A great surprise and a pleasant one, he brought choccies and flowers, we chatted along merrily for an hour or so. He then had to go a get some work done, after all he is an accountant, <u>so time is money!</u>

Emma came to start work on me and commenced with 20 minutes on trying to reactivate the receptors in my left foot then she switched to my shoulder blade/shoulder progressing down through my upper arm and elbow to my wrist/hand. When she had completed and hours work I was asked to stand, with Emma's help I stood and was coerced into an attempted walk with the walking stick. I managed a few dodgy paces then turned and did the same back............Good! That's enough for today

On Sunday my mate Peter popped in for a chat, he'd been Golfing again out near Barnsley way. Peter is as I have said before a joy to be with. It's just rubbish that we can't go and have a game of what we have done for decades, and that my friends is play League Table Tennis, well he can but I can't, not yet anyway.

Later Michael and Jon called and we had a trip up to Lidl, to get one or two more bits for Xmas. You never seem to buy all the things that are needed at this time of the year, but we try anyway.

Tuesday and the Ambulance arrive about 10:30hrs to take me to ARC. Once there it was have a cup of tea and watch the TV and wait until Alan came to take me through to the Gym. Alan came to collect me an hour later and first off was a lot of arm and leg stretches. I then progressed to walking tall with a quad stick whilst checking on my gait. This sometimes looked more like a crab walking than a bloke, but hey it was early days yet. Next job whilst walking between the parallel bars was "Look no Stick". Alan encouraged me to try walking between these bars with just the right hand in close proximity to a bar for surety. Not too bad but then again not too good either. Keep trying. No O.T. today.

We spent a QUIET Christmas Eve by ourselves preparing for the Big day. Our Denise & Bill, Michael & Jon and Jack joined us for Christmas Dinner. We didn't have to do anything. I did get loads of refreshments in, just in case! Whilst one family pair prepared all the meats the other pair did all the accoutrements. Our Jack as always did the dessert, something that he has done since his early teens, and he's twenty seven years old now, well done Grandson!

On Boxing Day the 26th I actual did my first walks with the Walking Stick. It is always dodgy and euphoric at the same time, just trying to master new skills. A quiet 34th Wedding Anniversary the day after but after a couple of days of activity i.e. all the family here for xmas and the new walking the day after, the 27th was a rest day.

On the 29th I had my first fall! I was hobbling past the settee and I must have not placed my foot in the correct place, therefore I fell on to the settee then slid partly down onto the floor. I did not hurt myself but remained on the floor but resting my upper body on the settee. We sent for the "City Wide Alarm Scheme" people to come and get me up. Twenty five minutes later they arrived, waddled my bottom onto this square rubber mat, plugged it into their compressor and pumped it full of air. It inflated little by little until I was in an excellent seating position and could with their help stand up and was then helped to my chair.

PANIC OVER!

Went to ARC on the 30th they were having a raffle and I won a box of Chocolates. Alan gave me a good stretch of both left arm and left leg and a little more walking between the parallel bars both with and without my walking stick. "Still standing" The R.A. (Rehab. Assistant) worked like a Trojan on the Muscles, Tendons, Fibres etc of my left hand and arm to help trigger a little more movement and then hopefully more use.

Another fairly quiet time on New Year's Eve, Maureen the neighbour popped in to see us as was usual in an afternoon. Worked my arm and leg with stretches and squats then we sat down and watched whatever was any good on the TV. Not much on that evening so Bed at about 10pm.

Same again New Year's day

Emma came on the 2nd Jan.2015 and then once weekly. Through January, February & March then because of costs we had to cut back to once fortnightly in April.

On Sunday 4th January 2015 we decided to order the lounge furniture that we had seen with Bill & Denise. Mike & Jon took us to Barker's, the furniture store, and we selected the colour, under advisement from the lads, to compliment our lounge. We ordered one Riser/Recliner chair for me, one 3 seat settee with a side operated leg/foot lift and a standard lounge chair. My chair was to be rushed though the factory and the others would take a few weeks.

On Tuesday at ARC Alan had me walking with my stick and tried to help me with my gait, which sometimes is a little crab like. No doubt this is because of my dropped foot and my over compensation not to catch the front part of the foot when walking and therefore lifting my hip. Do try it "you will look crab like as well". After the session I went to talk to this girl called Raquel whom I had been told had a mobility scooter going cheap. She told me how much she wanted for it and it was left at that for me think about! My old mate Gordon (ex of Oak Lane) came for his first call since he got let out, of said Rehab. Centre. His voice was still not working too well but he thinks it does as his wife can understand him, but we cannot at this stage of his vocal development.

Our Alan & Pauline called to see us on the Wednesday 7th January 2015 Stroke day plus 200, Emma came on Friday and worked as always very hard for me on my hand/arm/leg/walking with my stick. Helping me to find my correct foot placement and balance. She also worked on weight transference from one foot to the other and getting the weight over each hip in turn. This takes a long time in getting through to the brain as you are not confident about the weak leg and this takes many month's (well in my case it did) to conquer.

Well we had got our New Gates all looking lovely and all locked at nights so as to keep night prowler i.e. Thieves off of the Property, Guess what! The fence all down the side of the house/property got blown down in night time gale, Bloody great, just as I was starting to feel a little more secure and we are wide open to all and sundry. The following morning we rang the guy who did us the gates to ask for help, good man, he came down later, picked all the sections up off of the pavement, where they had blown onto and placed them on the garden. He asked whether we wanted him to get some new uprights and concrete to repair the fence. We got a price for the job and off he went. He came back on the Monday and got on with replacing the old fence supports that had rotted away with new ones, concreted them in place with the quick drying variety and attached the fence sections back in situ. Job complete by Lunch time.

A few weeks ago we made another attempt to have provided, a wheelchair, which I could use by myself. The answer was still NO! However, they would provide us with one which had a battery pack. This way Maureen would not have to push it around, just press the button for power assistance. Well today 13th of Jan. was the day that it arrived. This had to be pushed indoors as the battery power to the wheels was so strong that it would damage your carpets. The whole wheelchair attached with the Battery Pack was so heavy Maureen had problems just trying to push it indoors and it was for too heavy to lift over the back door threshold. This meant that it was of no use to her, the idea of the battery powered chair was to help not hinder her, we sent it back!. The same day at ARC was not too good either, as they were short staffed, so the time spent with Alan was severely limited so just a little arm/wrist stretching and foot to ankle stretching and bending but no walking, this time.

Emma came with a Jackie on Friday to see how things were going at home. Jackie is a head of Department at a Sheffield University and is a stroke arm rehabilitation specialist. Both she & Emma worked on the arm for about an hour. The whole lot was filmed to show the latest batch of Post graduate Students the techniques they needed to employ in the field.

We went out with Michael and Jon on Saturday, to Eden Mobility to look at Mobility Scooters, as I feel that I am now at a level that such a machine would be ideal for me, now that I can access my egress to the outside world, thanks to Phil and the pathway to my driveway gates.

More treats on Sunday18th Jan. Day 211.

My brother & sister-in-law came to take us out for a beer/wine. Alan had been checking out the pubs that I could access by wheelchair, with a disabled access toilet It was just smashing to be somewhere totally different for a change if only for a glass of beer and a chat. We only spent about an hour in the pub, but it was a whole new world for Maureen and me, after 7 months on the sidelines.

Spent a lot of time (or so it seemed) practicing the new style of walking that Emma & Alan had been showing me recently and my gait had certainly improved, according to Maureen, so it must be true and very accurate. You yourself can't tell whether things are getting better or not, you have to rely on your wife or partner, as these people are the ones that see you the most and know whether you are improving or need a quick kick up the rear end to get you going forward once more. Don't forget not just every day is a challenge but equally every hour can be as well, indeed every breath or step can be just as challenging.

Whilst away on rehab duty at the Assessment and Rehabilitation Centre ARC and continuing my rather good plodding. The friends that had loaned me the Riser/Recliner Chair came to take it away roughly one hour before my new one arrived. Loads of playing was done upon my return, i.e. just checking it out really!

On Thursday I actually went up stairs to change my trousers and went back down, mission accomplished, on my own!

Emma's visit on the Friday was accompanied by her mobile Plinth, which was set up in the lounge. I did not know that my leg could go in so many positions, it does now!. My foot moved itself very little but it was a bit of a first. This immediately followed the Gluteus work that Emma had just been doing. Maybe that's the secret, more buttock squeezes, Yippee!

On the 26th we took a taxi to another Mobility shop to check out their prices and stock. The Invacare Leo that was there was in my opinion just about the right size for more. It was also one of the 4mph footpath only types that I was interested in. The larger 8 mph types I thought were just too big and powerful at this stage in my recovery, maybe later!

However their prices were a little steep for me but at least I now knew what I was looking for!

I went to ARC on the Tuesday as per usual, when I went on to see Alan he fitted me up with a Functional Electrical Stimulation machine to see if my walking improved with the impulses that were fired down my leg to assist my foot to lift up. The first part of the system is attached by with two impulse carrying wires. The first One, which is of two wires/contacts pads, the top one you place at the head of the tibia and the other you place a couple of inches lower on the main muscle running down the length of the shin bone and the other, which is just of one contact is attached to an insole sited under your foot in the shoe/sandal/slipper, this one has a contact under your heel and this is the on/off switch. When the heel is firmly put down the impulses are curtailed but when not in floor contact the impulses begin. You control the strength of these impulses by turning the knob on the control unit, which is usually site on a waist belt or trouser pocket. This trial helped me with the walking, but felt strange until Alan re-adjusted the settings. Then he had me walking up and down the mini-stairs that they had for us to try out. I went up and down 3 times, I had a few problems with the left leg, always swinging across to the right-hand side, this happens a lot and until you can find some extra left leg control will continue to do so. At the end of this session Alan said that he would put me forward to the Northern General Hospital for my own FES system for my leg, as it had been quite a useful and successful exercise. At a later date he would also refer me for the Arm as well! After this I needed to go to the Loo, the nurse that wheeled me there gave me a bottle to use, so that they could check for any infection. It turned out that my Nitrates were up a little, but not unusual enough for an anti-biotics.

On Thursday 29th January 2015 Stroke day plus 222

I had a fell which was a loss of balance which was caused by this silly person trying to turn too quickly in the lounge and falling backwards. No problem I thought I am near to the wall, this will stop me going down! WRONG I did go down and hit the Jamb of the doorway, with the left side of my back. I was in fact a good two feet away from the wall and farther along it than I thought. I hit hurt my ribs and were sore for about 3 weeks. *I'll not do that in a hurry again!*

The next visit to see Alan at ARC he had me, with the FES in place, walking between the parallel bars up and over some wooden blocks, I could just about do it, but would need to practice more. Emma came on Friday with her Plinth and I had more of the leg pulls and pushes and some upper Arm work. Getting in at these fibres and sinews and tendons to get them thinking about trying to move a little more.

Ever since October 2014 when Mike & Jon purchased me a walking machine to help keep the circulation going in my legs and get them use to this action. I have used this machine daily and I would recommend one to anyone reading this Account of mine. The machine itself was a plug in device. You place a foot on each of two placements and switch on, these platforms would move forward and backwards and there are 2 speeds slow and very slow, but it does help.

You must try all things that are available, but still keep praying!

Sunday came and Mike & Jon took us to Macro, (a discount trade superstore). They needed some supplies for their Laundries and we saw and then bought a four camera security system. Which we got fitted a couple of weeks later by Jody a guy the family has used on many occasions.

Alan & Pauline came on the Monday and we went for pint & a chat at the Sportsman, Crosspool, a very Spartan amount of customers as you would expect for a Monday afternoon in February, but none the less, we enjoyed visiting somewhere different and talking about what was next on my Agenda. Alan said that he was constantly looking around for alternative venues that we could visit where they could get me in and who had an easy to get to and use, wheelchair accessible toilet. Lots of Pubs, Restaurants have these Disabled toilets but they are not always "Easy Accessible".

On Tuesday at ARC I made an agreement to buy the Mobility Scooter off of the Lady that was selling a "Shoprider" for £150 I knew that it would not be a superb example of a Scooter but not knowing anything about these, agreed to call at her house on the following Sunday, and if it was in a reasonable condition, would buy it.

Until you have been to a recognized NHS Rehab Centre you cannot assess your own situation. You soon find out that if you can talk, maybe move in a controlled way, whilst in your wheelchair, have good recognisance and have a good general state of Health, you are bloody lucky, because most stroke survivors do not!. Apart from not having poor arm and or leg movement the biggest problem that you notice is the ability to be able to speak and be understood. This is very frustrating for both the person talking and others trying to work out what they are saying. Whilst going to ARC I had many a conversation with Gordon and just occasionally you got the idea of what he was talking about. Gordon was obviously going there for speech therapy as he did not suffer as much as others there with limb problems.

Just the foot drop................mind you that is bad enough on its own!

Jane from the Stroke Association came to visit on Wednesday and after updating us on ALL stroke stuff, courses she was running both shortly and in the fear future, said she would put us forward to be able use the Community Transport, a part of the Local Passenger Transport services. A service you collected and later brought back to your home. They operate within the city boundaries with just one or two exceptions. You had a small amount to pay for each usage.

The Furniture store phoned to say that the other ordered furniture and arrived and could be delivered on between 11 – 12am next Wednesday. This was exactly how we wanted things as we had to contact a Charity to come and collect our existing furniture that needed to be removed, to create the necessary space for them. We managed to get hold of Oxfam and they agreed to come between 10- 11 am, an hour before the new stuff arrived.

When Emma arrived on Friday she brought her Plinth in with her. First I had to stand with my back touching it, then sit on the edge then get on a lie on my side, with Emma's help . She could then begin work on my stroke affected left arm and shoulder but mainly the subluxed shoulder. Fortunately I get very little pain, which believe me is wonderful, it was not always like this, especially in Oak Lane, but things seemed to have settled down a lot these last few months.. Emma brought with her a balance pad. This was about 20 inches square and roughly 3 inches thick of compressed rubber. The idea was that I would stand on this at my back kitchen window and practice sideways movements & squats, whilst having the worktop to hold onto if needed. I found this to be very useful indeed. I always had good balance, due to all the sport that I had played, but it certainly did give me more movement options stood where I did at this window.

On the morning of the 14th February, St.Valentines day I walked up & down stairs. This must have been my first up & down because I made a note about it in my Diary, so bully for me. On the Sunday Michael & Jon came to takes us up to look at this Mobility Scooter, we rang the Lady first to check that all was still okay for our visit. Upon arrival the Scooter was on her forecourt, she came out of the house to join us. First I had a little go then Jon, all seemed in good working order, it wasn't the prettiest scooter in town, but as a starter one, would suffice. That night it poured down all night, the following day when I took the scooter for it's first run-out in the Park, it struggled to hold charge, even though we had had it on charge since we got back home with it. We had Jody come and set up the outside all-weather sockets, 10 days before this purchase. We had been totally naïve about needing to protect the scooter from the elements and had therefore ruined the power pack, but instead of getting new batteries and throwing more money at this scooter decided to buy a new one and have this one scrapped.

Tuesday the 17th February 2015 Stroke day plus 241.

At Arc we continued on from the last session, that of walking in between the rails and stepping up & down off the blocks. Still having problems controlling my left leg swing, but working on it! The day after Oxfam came as requested and took away our lovely leather 3 piece suite, once they had gone the new Suite arrived and with in being just a little smaller was more easily brought in to the house and sited. My wife was eager to try out the settee with the leg lift control, it really has been a wonderful purchase for us both.

Emma came again on Thursday, she was straight into action, onto the floor, my shoe and sock was off in seconds, so it seemed, and Emma was working the fibres, receptors, tendons, muscles etc. of my foot and lower leg.

By feeling scratching tickling and manipulating, she hoped that I would get some movement, hopefully one day!

Phil came on Thursday as requested to finalize the Scooter Plinth that he was laying for us outside our back kitchen window, adjacent to the pathway that he had laid. The concrete came and was laid on the Friday, but we would obviously have to keep off of it until dried. Phil came back on the Monday and laid some edging bricks on the newly laid concrete plinth as a boundary for my future scooter(s) safety.

ARC Tuesday was just some arm massage by the Rehab Assistant and a short spell of walking, I told Alan that I was going to the Sheffield Hallam University to assist Emma Richards the following week, as she had asked me if I would join her and others for Hallam University's Post Graduate Physiotherapists' "Patient Assessment" as part of their Masters Degree Course.

Went to the Parkhead Tavern with A & P on Monday 25th February, we enjoyed our chats, beers and coffee's, cheers Alan. The Parkhead is quite good to access with the wheelchair and they also have Disabled parking places. We always enjoy our family chats with Alan & Pauline, keeping ourselves up to date on who was doing what or where they had gone etc.

CHAPTER 13 / Day 250

THURSDAY . February 26th 2015

My first visit to the FES clinic, based in the Mobility & Rehab centre of the Northern General Hospital, was to see a lady called Jill who gave me this control box and some stick-on patches, which you put in different positions on your arm for different movements, I was to use this Fes control twice for 10 minutes each day and then increase gradually day by day up to two 30 minute sessions per day. Hopefully this would give you some increased movement with the hand and fingers. I also had my grip strength tested, I managed to pull 6kg first time then 8kg on the second go. I thought, not bad! But I don't know what Jill thought. She told me that she would get in touch with ARC for them to send a leg referral on my behalf, as she could not help me with my leg until such a referral had arrived from them requesting this treatment for my leg.

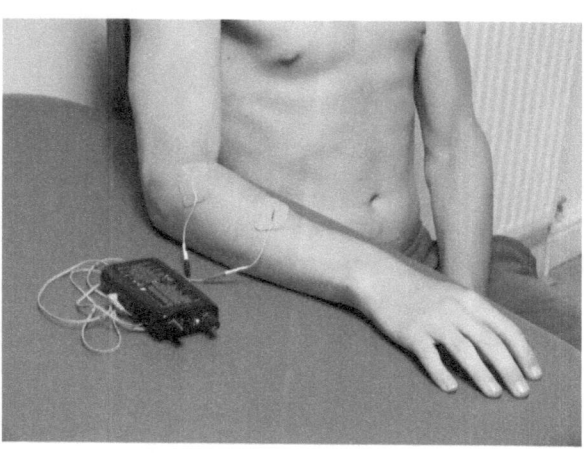

We went up to Clarke & Partners on the Friday to check out theirs "Special Offers" on Mobility Scooters. They had an Invacare Leo in at half price so I ordered the blue one immediately, as this was the make & model that I had been fancying for a while. The delivery was agreed, late afternoon next Thursday 05/03/15.

The week of Sheffield Hallam University Post Grads. MSC Course.

This Course was to take place at the Robert Winston building of the Collegiate Campus of the University. Robert M. L. Winston also formally known as Lord Professor Winston. **FMedSci, FRSA, FRCP, FRCOG, FIBiol, FREng**, is and has been the Chancellor of the University since 5th October 2001.

I went on Monday, Tuesday, Thursday & Friday. I would be collected at 12:15 on each of these days and returned home by 3pm.

On the Monday I met my "Students" Maryam & Nada. Maryam is from Cairo and Nada from Muscat in Oman. Two very intelligent professional young Ladies, who used their skills to assist my left limbs to recover a little bit more and look after me, during these four days.

The first day was purely an assessment day. i.e. Find out what my arm & leg were capable of, and what sort of sensors were present in them. Tuesday and the emphasis was firmly on my weaker left leg. After about three quarters of an hour of massage & manipulation, I actually walked a few yards without any aids. This was a first and one that I am still trying to improve upon, both in the quality of walking and the distance. On Thursday my two Arabian Ladies worked on both my arm & leg simultaneously. Whilst Nada manipulated my leg, ankle and foot, Maryam worked my hand, wrist, elbow & shoulder. Then they combined to try and free-off my shoulder blade, which seems to prefer not to move, their success at this was very limited. *But it will move eventually, come what may!*

Friday was Arm Day and the whole class was there to watch Senior Lecturer Jackie Hammersley work on my arm whilst discussing the said arm with the class within a sort of Question and Answer scenario. My arm thought that this was a wonderful time to relax and enjoy itself whilst getting the best of all worlds from Jackie and the floor. We even had Gerry Scott join us, another Senior Lecturer, who has vast experience and who also specializes in upper limb recovery. Gerry of course is the Physiotherapist that had put me in touch with Emma, in the first place. I was sad that the week was over, It is always good to receive specialist input from other highly qualified Physiotherapists as well as your regular Physio.

On Monday, 9th March I received an appointment letter for the FES Clinic for my leg, which had now got referred by Alan at ARC, this he confirmed when I was there the day after. We arrived at the Hospital on the Wednesday, early for my 12:30hr appointment. I was asked to walk alongside Amanda who was to see me today. We entered their room with cameras set up in many positions. This place was geared to assessing Stroke Victims walking abilities, the room floor is marked with distance markers to see and record just how fast/slow you could walk over a straight 12 yard distance both with & without a walking aid. I was then told that as far as she was concerned the FES would be an advantage to me and I was issued with the control machine, some stick-on patches and an instruction book on how to use the machine and where to place the contacts electrodes. I was sure that without the book, I would forget all that I had been told and instructed to do, with regard to this piece of equipment.

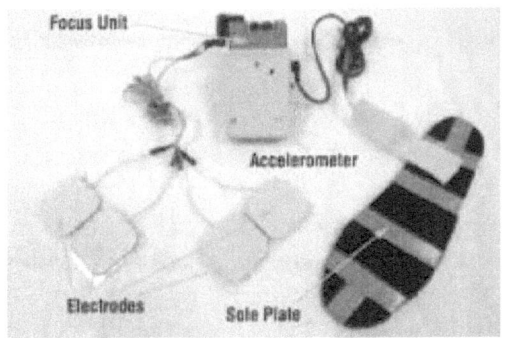

Thanks for the book, as I had forgotten by the time we had got home and needed to revise all of this information. After a period of 4/5 months the FES had created a sore patch on my leg. I had been using this equipment every day for my walking and it had helped my gait quite a lot. However in our opinion it wasn't assisting any long term betterment of the foot drop. So with the sore patch on my leg and the ongoing impulses sent down this leg we decided to leave it alone, if only to let the skin recover from the damage caused.

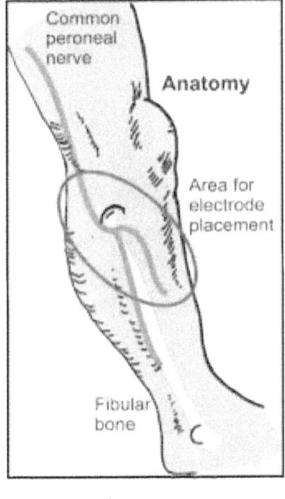

We had a trip to an out of Town Shopping Centre in York with Bill & Denise on the Saturday. Nice change to get out of my home town for a change and just see something different, even if it was only the

Motorway and A roads there and back. Denise had researched the shopping centre and ordered a mobility scooter for me to use, when we got there. The only thing we had to do on arrival was go to this shop and leave my wheelchair behind as surety against the scooter. Good thinking Denise! It really was very handy and gave me greater independence around the shops. I even bought a weatherproof jacket whilst there!

On the 19th March it was back to the Hallam Uni, this time it was Maryam & Nada's presentation of their Roger Turner's case Studies to their Tutors and the other Physiotherapists on this Course. Alan from ARC came along to see and experience all the various variations that would be presented that day. As all other participants would in turn give their presentations to the floor just like Maryam & Nada had done with me.

To assist with a more upright walking gait I had ordered a pair of Hiking Poles, these arrived on Saturday21st March. They took a little getting used to, but I felt that these would be better for me "Long Term". I have not been disappointed in them at all and would recommend them to other survivors of Strokes.

CHAPTER 14 / Day 277

WEDNESDAY. MARCH 25th 2015

DRIVER ASSESSMENT DAY.

This was the day that I had been longing for, for the past 277 days.

Maureen & I took a Taxi up to Lightwood House the HQ of the NHS Physiotherapy in Sheffield. We entered and the lady in the reception area talked to us and together we filled in some forms, Personal Stuff. Then she talked me through the system for the Driving Assessment, once satisfied that we understood what would happen. She took me through into the next Office to meet the Assessor/Examiner.

He seemed a very pleasant chap and soon made me feel relaxed about the whole experience, that was about to happen.

We went outside, I was in my wheelchair, so was pushed around to the drivers door, where I stood up to access the car. I got into the car the Assessor gave me full instructions about the controls and told how to use them, both the hand ones and how to use the foot accelerator and brake. Fortunately I had driven an Automatic car before so no problems there. The hand joystick control I found was the better of the two type of hand unit that he let me use. Before we started to drive, both my wife & I thought that I would be driving around their enclosed compound. Nothing could have been further from the truth. We set off and the Assessor, whom we will call Bill, said drive to the main Road, turn right at the top and proceed forward.

About half a mile Bill said turn right on to the Basegreen Estate. We went around and around this Estate, turning left, turning right, going down and up gradients. Once satisfied that I had mastered these maneuvers we set course for another Area, this was the Crystal Peaks Shopping Centre a very busy area with lots of traffic and loads of Roundabouts to encounter. Ten or twelve roundabouts later and about one hour into this drive, Bill told me to "Lets make our way back to Base", this took another 15 minutes or so and "Just park it over there" was the instruction from Bill. When this was complete we went back to his Office, Bill said "Well Done". An excellent drive but before you drive we would advise 2 or 3 Lessons with a specialist Driving School to just hone your skills. You will be hearing from us in a few weeks! We ordered a taxi to take us back home at the opposite side of the City.

We received the Driving Assessment Report about 3 weeks later and to my surprise receive my New Driving License, for Automatic & Adapted cars only about a month later. What a lovely surprise this was as neither my wife nor I was expecting this to happen.

The following Tuesday at ARC they had me walking about 200/250 yards in Total which was very satisfying but equally very tiring as well. It certainly is mentally a lot easier to walk with someone with good expertise of patient safety, knowledge of their problems/weaknesses and the strength of body to give patients peace of mind. With that comes the confidence to tackle whatever is being asked of them, for you to do. Emma had been coming weekly up to this point but because of costs alas, had to cut calls back to fortnightly. This would also give me more time to practice what I had learned from her, regarding my walking.

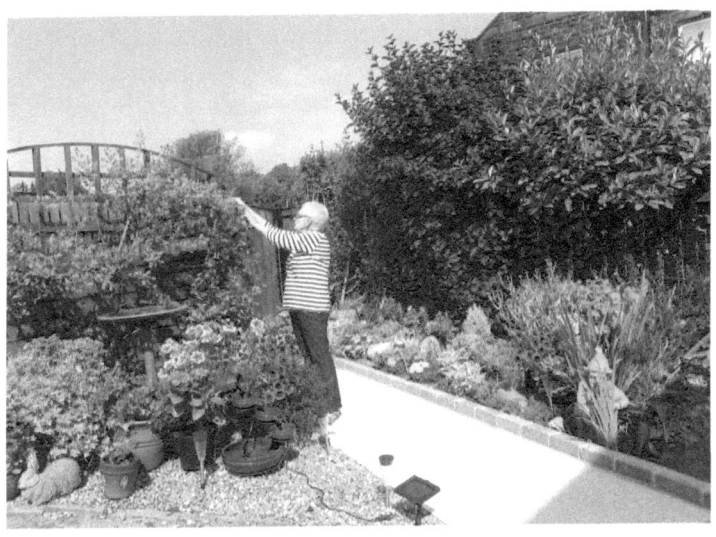

Easter Sunday 5th April 2015 was a lovely warm sunny day. I was walking up my Garden Path heard a noise turned just slightly, but a little too fast, and lost balance. I landed on my well padded bottom in the space as shown above, between where my wife's feet are and the light sensor, onto the pebbled area.

I thought "What a daft thing to do". As I have said I am well padded in that area of my anatomy so no pain or discomfort was felt. Just stupidity! I did knock the odd plant out of the way and tip over the Bird bath, but no lingering problems. However I needed to send for the City Wide Alarm people to get me upright once more. Two minutes later our Michael rang to enquiry how I was, as City Wide had phoned to ask if they were near by, as CW were short of staff, this being Easter day. Michael was on a weekend break up Yorkshire, so no was their answer.

Another 10 minutes passed and an Emergency Ambulance arrived as they had been summoned. They could see that I was okay and just needed getting up. The ambulance Lady just bent over and pulled me upright………..Wow!   They said that the alarm people often ring them when under Personnel shortage.

Just for the Record. Easter Monday 06/04/2015 reached 20degrees C.

April 8th and I actually assisted with a bit of Gardening, just a little digging and prodding with my 4 pronged earth agitator. Power it down, with my good arm, into the hardened soil and rotate back U& forth to loosen said soil. Then Maureen could do a little planting of new Flower bulbs with their roots. You know the ones that are sold in DIY stores that have just started to grow a little. Take them home, take them out of their pots and plant in the garden, easy. The lads came down and sorted out some rocks to position for our new rockery, it looks good as well! The following Monday Our Al took us around a Garden Centre so we could get a few more plants for the garden.

Tuesday 14th Alan had me walking all around ARC today. Slowly and with rests, I made the 150yards in about 15 minutes. Gosh that was tiring!

After this I went in to see Doctor Ali and he administered Botox to my weak sided Arm & Leg, a total of 15 injections. I hope these work I could do with finding the starter button for my arm especially………They did not give me any improvement in my arm or leg at all.

What a disappointment!

CHAPTER 15 / Day 299

16th April 2015

I had seen on the TV News recently about a very seriously injured Paratrooper by the name of Ben Parkinson, who had started having Hyper Baric Treatment in the hope of assisting his mobility. The TV account said that it seemed to be having a big help for Ben. So I thought about this and decided to ask my Consultant about the possible help it could be to me. He did not know whether it would help me or not but if I was going to try it out could I report back to him with my thoughts/results. I gave me the go-ahead to try this treatment if I so desired. I searched around for a Hyper Baric Chamber and discovered that there was on at the M.S. Centre at Catcliffe. A Hyper Baric Chamber is a Decompression Chamber that allows the controller to regulate the pressure within, Just like saving a diver that has surfaced too fast and has "The Bends" It is about 12 feet in external diameter and roughly 10 internally. I has seating for about maybe 8 people, at a pinch. It is made of steel and the door is multi-locked when re-compression or de-decompression takes place. The door is only open at "One Atmoshere"

I rang them up to enquire about the possibility of me trying this out. The answer was of course I can use it but I would have to pay an annual membership fee of £15 to the M.S. Centre first, this I did and was booked in for my first go on Thursday 16th.

Thursday came and over we went to the Centre via the Community transport. Logged in at the reception area and told to wait whilst my time was due. At 1pm the door of the Chamber opened and a gentleman took control of the situation. First he assisted the four of us that had booked this journey into compression into our seats, within. We were each helped with on with our breathing apparatus; he then left to control the compression ratio from his control post. Because this was my first time, we were only taken down to one half Atmosphere of pressure. The air was gradually expelled from the chamber whilst you received pure oxygen through your nose & mouth apparatus. When muscles get neat oxygen, it apparently aids their speedier recovery. I assume that is why lots of Professional footballers use this method.

The noise of this really took some getting used to, as the compression setting was attained. This took about 10 minutes and was then maintained for a further 45 minutes. I sat reading the Kindle e-reader that I had taken with me for this purpose. I was breathing heavily to get maximum benefit from my experience in the chamber but it was very boring and the time dragged by, but that did not matter if it was doing me some good. At the end of our period in this Chamber the air pressure was increased back up to one Atmosphere, so at not to give us the bends, i.e. Decompression Sickness (air bubbles that can get into your blood and could pain, cramp or breathing difficulties or worse).

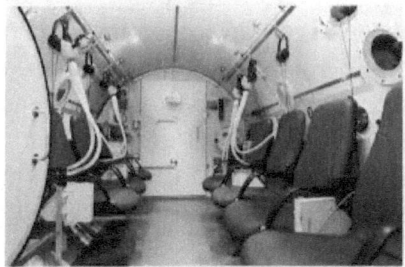

When the session was complete the door was opened by the Controller and I went to talk to Maureen about my experience and book for another session for in a couple of week's time. The bus arrived shortly to take us home. After our initial membership payment the Chamber cost was only £6 per session, cheap or what! An experience that I would whole heartedly recommend to all Stroke survivors who do not have any residual medical problems that could be made worse with decompression. **<u>Check with your Doctors first</u>** About 10 days after going in the Chamber I had an attack of Labyrinthitis, I problem I had had a couple of years beforehand but thought that I was completely cured of. Labyrinthitis is an infection/fluid within the canals of the inner ear and causes you to have very severe balance problems... Now that is probably one of the last problems you need when having walking and balance problems from the stroke as well. When I first had this manifest itself, I woke up one morning and I suddenly felt that I was turning 90 degrees, whilst lying on my back, and about to fall out of bed. For those that can remember the "Whirling Pit" situation that one could into after a long nights drinking session. Then this was much worse! I attempted to stand up but just fell back on the bed. This is where I stayed for the next couple of days until this initial attack had subsided. There is no cure for this illness and it is just something that will first ease off then just go away. Usually with 5/7 weeks. Mine lasted 5 months then it came back again a few months later for a couple of weeks then I got freed from its grasp. Until, that is, the Decompression brought it back a little, but just a little when you have had a Stroke is scary, very **Scary!**

On Wednesday the 22nd April 2015 I was taken to play Table Tennis at the Shiregreen Working Mens Club by some friends who ran their League Club out of this venue. (In fact it was the place where the final stage scenes for The Full Monty film were performed). This was my first game for a year, but this time I was *sat having a go* in my wheelchair. Awkward, bloody awkward to say the least, but after a 10 minute knock up, my timing started to return and I actually gave my opponent a little bit to think about, I played five games that evening. After, the lads patted me on the back and said that I had in fact done better than one of the other lads that had a TIA a couple of years before and who still suffered a bit during matches. When you practice, you tend to play more contracted and patterned play, In matches you play a more cunning and deconstructed game to surprise and confuse your opponent. This is when the Trained Brain needs to be at its most astute and sharp and the body at its most controlled and yet flexible state of awareness. What a good night it was, getting back to a little more normality! I got home about 10pm. *Knackered but happy!*

23rd April Went to Northern General today and saw Alison who gave the FES for my upper limb (arm) this was to facilitate the movement in my fingers/wrist and also to help straighten my arm at the elbow. The day after Emma came as usual, once a fortnight. I walked up & down the staircase twice and this too was a FIRST.

My diary states **"A GREAT WEEK."**

CHAPTER 16 / Day 310

MONDAY. APRIL 27th 2015

Monday 27th Our Chiropodist Mark came and cut my toe & finger nails.

Tuesday ARC Alan keeps me hard at the walking whilst trying to free –up the arm,

Wednesday Specsavers man came to re-test my eyes after the previous errors that he made.

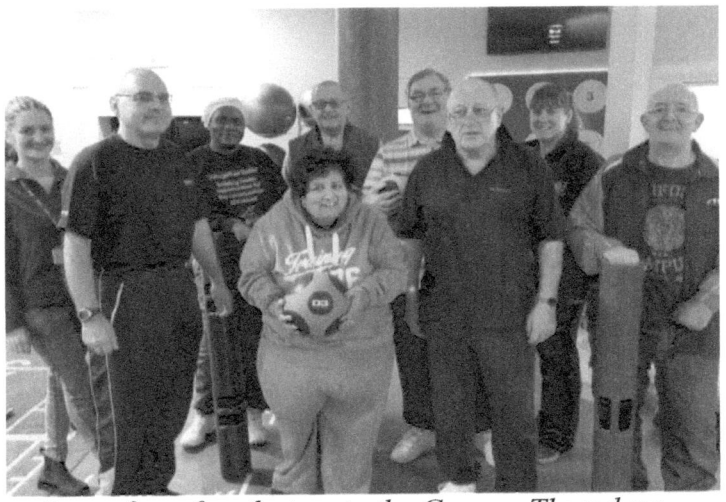

Just a few of us that go to the Gym on Thursdays.

Thursday came and it was a biggy I did not realize it at the time but it changed my life for the better. Community Transport came and took both Maureen & myself down to Ponds Forge Gymnasium. To join up with other Stroke Survivors that went to the Stroke Gym run by Lucy Annandale the referral Coach, Lucy helps and assists all she can to allow you to use the specialized equipment that is at our disposal. There is an area where these machines form an ovoid shape, which you work around, clockwise. You spend 5 minutes on each piece of equipment. We met with Jane Hammond the Stroke Association's representative for Sheffield who in turn introduced us to Lucy.

My first time today at Ponds Forge, thanks to Lucy I did a lot more than I thought that I could do!

Friday we went out with Alan &Pauline, I enjoy these times as I can just relax and have a good chin-wag, a glass of beer and discuss the week that has just gone and what indeed is cropping up in the near future.

At ARC on 5th May Dr. Ali administered Botox (<u>Botulinum toxin</u>) to my lower left leg, let me just say if this assists in my ability to control any or all movements, as I still suffer from high toning in my leg, I can only say its bloody slow at getting started, Maybe I should just use it to get rid of some wrinkles. However, this toning is not as bad as in my left arm and my Pectoral muscles thereof. Maybe one day this will help but if it does, I can only say its bloody slow at getting started. Alan had me walking outside again, but the other way around the building, getting better at this! Then John arrived to take me home as was usual at the end of each of these sessions by NHS Ambulance, this usually took 25mins. If we left by say 3:10 but any later and it was a good hour, because by then the schools were coming out and that as we all know is when millions of Mothers hit the streets in their 4 x 4's hit and block the streets, sometimes!

Maureen & I went on a trip out to Crystal Peaks via the Community Transport this cost us a total of £16 return. By going this way I could take along my Mobility Scooter and this is a godsend to getting about and having that wonderful feeling of Independence. I get to follow Maureen into the shops and around the Market and in the lift to go down to other shops and eats places, then we can call for Lunch in one of the Restaurants. It's good to be able to do this.

The rest of May was pretty much as most months would be. The main difference was that Emma got me walking by putting my right foot forward first then out stepped by my left and repeated until you could call it a walk. With this is in all walking you have to have faith in the weak leg, to be able to support you, it takes a lot of time and effort to master this. June was "same old" that is to say; it followed the same path as May did, Emma, ARC, Crystal Peaks, & Gym. On Saturday 20th June, Michael & Jon took us on a little trip to Matlock, that wonderful Spa town in North Derbyshire. The weather was not particularly good but we enjoyed the trip enormously. They came back the following day along with Annabell for Fathers Day.

The last two weeks of June was the only time that I actually got brave enough to go without my wheelchair. This meant that once the Ambulance arrived at home to collect me, then it was down to my legs to do the work. Upon arrival at ARC I had to walk to a seat in the lounge, a distance of 40 yards or thereabouts and henceforth, when called, into the Gym to see Alan. Kay worked on my upper left limb whilst Alan tried, yet again, to stretch my Achilles tendon, to help facilitate me in getting my heal on the floor more easily.

Monday 29th June 2015. Day 373. We had agreed to go to a place called "Paces" This is school in the north of the City that help disabled children to better their lives. We went to meet up with representatives from the Peto Institute. An organization that had been doing a different style of Rehabilitation exercise programme for many years in Hungary & Romania, predominantly with children. They had started to use this programme down on the UK's south coast on Adults with various results, and decided to try to branch out up North.

The course they were trying to sell us was one of ten weeks of twice weekly 2.5 hour sessions at £10 per time. Some attendees from the 29th Junes meeting signed up. I was a little sceptical so decided against this on this occasion but not until I had been back for an assessment. I was not too keen on what I was told at this assessment but thought I'll wait until I've got some feed back about this first course before scrapping the idea all together. The feed back that I have subsequently received is one of mixed feeling as to its usage in any form of adult recovery. So maybe someday, maybe never!

Tuesday saw me go to ARC but without my wheelchair. This was so that I had to concentrate purely on my walking as in, all the time I was there and back into my home upon return. More practice makes perfect, well it doesn't in my case, but it is bound to improve me, if only by 0.001% on each of these occasions.

I will no doubt get to do more and more as time goes on. This is my hope, and I am sure that I will be proved right in the long run. The following day I had to go to the Medical Rehabilitation Centre at the Northern General Hospital for an FES update, they needed to see me walking and make any necessary adjustments to my Control box settings. They decided that my walking was coming on just fine, if any layman who saw me would certainly not agree but who are these laymen and what do they know anyway. My walking was improving bit by bit but I would not be contesting Usain Bolt to any form of race in the near or distant future. His loss not mine.. He! He!

No alterations to the Control Box were made, maybe next time..

The following Tuesday 7th July 2015 S.D. plus 381. at ARC I saw both Alan & Kay the O.T. they both did a little work on both my Arm and Leg plus a little walk between the parallel bars with the up and over the different heighted boxes. Then it was "Well Roger you can carry on coming for another week or two but we cannot really help you to recover any better than you are at this moment and others need to have the opportunity to come here." I said that I would finish with immediate effect and give others a chance to come for their assistance in the recovery process. In all fairness I had not improved a lot in recent weeks and any further advancements made would be of the long and laborious types. ***"little by little by little by little by little"*** *as the old Dusty Springfield song stats......Must have referred to something like Stroke recovery or losing someone you love!*

Brother Alan and his wife took us down town to the Famous Frog & Parrott bar on Division Street, Sheffield 1. 'tis a good place to spend an hour or two people watching but within the bar and the Students in their variety of clothing and footwear and indeed Make-up and hairstyles. Great watching indeed!. Went to the Gym. as usual on the Thursday, this does me the power of good!, When Emma came on Friday she asked me how I found the Balance Pad after the four months or so since she had brought it for me to practice with. I told her that it wasn't used a lot but occasional use was helpful. I kept it for another couple of months before returning it back to Emma to assist another survivor or ailing client.

Sun bathing, sat on my Mobility Scooter on our Scooter Pad or off to the Gym or out with Alan & Pauline or Mike & Jon or Denise & Bill or around the park or to the shops was how July went past. That is until the 27th when we had an appointment to go to the Orthotics dept. at the Northern General Hospital. We had this appointment to see Connor one of the specialists at this Dept. We arrived and I was given a leg splint this was a strapping for the leg, another for the foot and an elasticated section to attach between them which would hopefully lift the dropped foot sufficient to be able to walk better without the FES being attached. FES is often considered by some not all but some not to be the *"Be all and end all"* of assistance for this affliction.(If that is what you can call it) I still use this today as I find it better then FES, only because FES and its continual electrical impulses gets to you after a while.. Not much happened then until the 10th August when we went out with Alan & Pauline on his Birthday. Stroke Day plus 415 We did the usual sort of stuff but these are very special afternoons for both me & Maureen. Its not just the meeting but more the getting out and doing things that are quite normal and being able to hear other different voices, see other trees and houses and just a general look around. Must of us just notice what we want to notice. Look a little longer and take in the views more. You will find that there is so much more that you normally miss. More beauty, more information and loads and loads of pleasure, simple pleasure, the sort you often just take for granted such as the Bird's singing and the flora & fauna that lies abundant everywhere you look. Not a lot happened again for a few days and then I met an old Table Tennis Team mate from 20 years ago. He was now playing for the same club that I had been playing for until that fateful day back in 2014. Neil ask me to go and have a knock (a friendly game) at the Wadsley Bridge Club, which is not at Wadsley Bridge but in fact Malin Bridge. We agreed to meet up on Friday 21st August at 1p.m. This we did and we played (well he played and I attempted to play) a few games. The first practice 15 minutes were atrocious, I had all on just hitting the ball. However when we got into game play I started to get some good stuff back, but found this a hard task sat in my wheelchair. i.e. a totally different height than I would have been if I had in fact been able to stand and play, but you do become accustomed to this new if not improved position and your game gets better the more you play. After an hour and a half, we finished, I thanked Neil for picking me up and helping me onto this new step on my recovery slope. We had both decided that we should join Shiregreen T.T. club, we gave them a call and we got an invitation to meet the for a Knock on the following Wednesday @ 7p.m. Neil said that he would pick me up and bring me back home afterwards, mmm sounds good to me!.

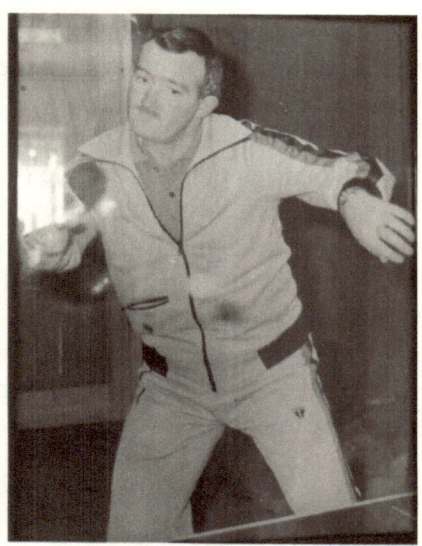
Me in bygone days

On Sunday Mike & Jon picked Maureen & myself up to take us for Lunch. We settled on the really nice fish Restaurant called Whitby's where it was agreed that we would also meet up with Annabell & William. It really is good to see these two having an enjoyable and relaxing time. The kids were brought and collected later by their mother.

The Cod & Chips there are really top quality and I wholeheartedly recommend their restaurant to anybody who likes this food. It is a large Plaice or is that Place but the service is superb and not costly, for the quality that you receive.

On Tuesday 25th July SD +430 August Paul from the Stroke Association called in to give us come information on up and coming events. The one that I was interested in was a six or was it an eight week course that incorporated lots of different sports to try out such as Boccia, Indoor bowls and Table Tennis.

Paul said that he would be arranging the Community Transport to pick all of us that wanted to go up every week. A few days before week one, we had a ring from the transport people to say it was not possible to take us to the Venue. Which for me, was across the City at Handsworth. I then text Jane the Stroke co-ordinator to say that the Venue was too far away and therefore too costly for me to get there by Taxi, so alas I would not be attending but would look forward to any other of these courses that were more local to Hillsborough, my area of Sheffield. I have not yet heard of any more of these courses, but you never know!

Wednesday came, Neil arrived and off we went to play some "Ping Pong" at the Shiregreen club. We arrived, Neil went in to tell them that we had arrived. The guys there opened up a side door to the playing area, on the other side of the building, where I could gain better access and indeed better egress after the playing was done.

My first session was against Chris, a man I had known for the best part of 40 years, every since he was a teenager. Chris was kind and gentle with me at first, until he realized that even if I had certain playing problems. After 10 minutes I got used to the pace and spin and as long as Chris played into my *"Gold Zone"* then I could give him a decent game. Chris is vastly experienced and has played in Sheffield Top division for a lot of years, even if at the moment the team he plays for is in the second division. He won the one game that we played 11 – 8. Next I played Gary maybe not as good as Chris but generally more ruthless. (After all he is an Accountant)

Ha! Ha! He beat me 11 – 4 I then played three more of the guys before it was time to call it a day and head for my bed. Neil enjoyed his night there as well. He took me home and we agreed to go back for more, the following week. We also decided to go back for another session at the old club. The next trip up to Shiregreen went pretty much as the first session but there was one or two different players this time, so we got to play other different styles and standards.

Emma came and we had a great work out on my foot and arm and I practiced my walking. I mentioned that I was considering Acupuncture for my Spastic arm and what did she think of this. Emma said that she was not sure whether it would be any good for me or not. If you want to try it, it is up to you Rog..................Still considering.   Emma however did give me the name and number of a very good Physio that also a practicing Acupuncturist. The day before at Pond's Forge Gym. I had been given some info. About a new form of Gym. which is being run by Gavin Church, a physiotherapist that I knew of from my Rehabilitation Centre days. I said that I would ring Gavin, whose number Lucy had given to me, and enquire about the Gym, he was running. Gavin told me that it was to be an eight weeks course, twice weekly on Tuesday & Thursday afternoons for about an hour a time. The course was limited to a maximum of 6 participants. It would not cost anything at all but needed all participants to give at least 85% attendance. The sponsors of the course who would be keeping an eye closely on the results, was Sheffield Hallam University Physiotherapy Department.

This new type of Gym. which had come over from Americas west coast was called *"CROSSFIT*

TRAINING' It was all about weights and balance combined, i.e. could Stroke survivors manage the movement with weights and how easy was it for them with continually increased weights with this movement. The Course's time scale was 29th September until 30th November, the last session being the Courses Assessment day.

> The Stroke class was set up 2years with the help and support of the Stroke Association. Its aim is to support and aid in the rehabilitation of individuals after a stroke. They come with a variety of conditions and impairments that make main stream exercise difficult to access so these classes offer that stepping stone back into exercise and improve their daily living. The first class focuses on a single exercise concept, for example Bending, Pulling, Pushing, Locomotion etc. Participants in this class tend to have impaired mobility, limited function in one or more limbs. The other classes is based on similar exercises done as a circuit with access to the main gym as a progression.
>
> When we first launched the classes they were isolated in a separate space, but over the past 2 years I have found doing these classes in the gym has broken down some of the barriers and helped individuals feel apart of the ordinary hustle and bustle of a gym. This has given many the confidence to become members, thereby enabling them to train on their own.

Roger is a very committed gentleman. I have been impressed by his determination. He worked with me for several months before taking part in a project run by a physio friend of mine – Gavin Church. I visited this project a few weeks before it completed and was surprised to see how this work has changed Roger. There was a massive difference in him, his demeanour and his mobility. This transformation in Roger inspired me to emulate Gavin's work in the first of my Stroke classes. Roger continues to go from strength to strength supporting and inspiring others in the class.

Lucy Annandale
Exercise Referral Coordinator

CHAPTER 17 / Day 448

Saturday September 12th 2015

Maureen and I had decided a few weeks ago that we needed to try taking a Holiday abroad. Our choice was Benidorm on the Costa Blanca in Spain. A destination that we know of through various holidays that we had taken there over the years. I thought that with it being our first holiday since my Stroke that maybe we needed it sorting by a specialist company. We also know that the Resort caters for the old or disabled through the mobility hire shops available there along with got overall facilities within the Resort. I got prices in from first, Disability Access Holidays and then from Enable Holidays for Hotels that were recommended in their brochures as having adapted rooms and poolside assistance etc. The cost did not vary much at all, the difference was about £15 in total. So with that we booked with D.A.H. the holiday was for 10 days from Manchester Airport to Alicante Airport, this being the nearest to our destination Resort.

Mike & Jon took us to the Airport on departure day. We were flying with Jet2 so had to find out how to find them check in our Luggage and then go to the Help desk for Airport assistance. Once we got there the Staff member of staff at the desk said that he would send for someone to take us through to the plane, Mike & Jon left us waiting!

Forty minutes later we ask where the guy was that was taking us to our plane as time was passing by, the flight was due to leave in three quarters of an hour. They could not find the assistance man designated to take us through to our plane. It turns out that had taken another wheelchair bound man to his flight instead. They instructed another assistant to take us immediately. Whilst awaiting this man to arrive, we found out that the original guy had clocked off and gone home or caught a plane to ?. Who knows where! He was not seen again that day at least.

The second / replacement Aircraft assist turned up within roughly 8 minutes and off we went to our dispatch zone via police & customs control., afterwards we just managed to grab a sandwich for the flight before being rushed through to the awaiting plane. We were transferred onto the loading vehicle with the hydraulic lift. Up we went at the plane we had to walk across a small footbridge to enter the plane at the front, sort of opposite where the other passengers would have gained access to the seating zone.

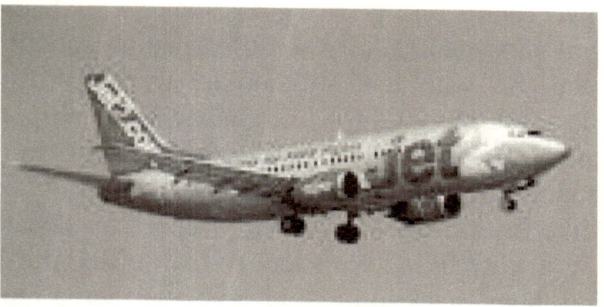

Once we had entered the plane, I was helped into my seat in Row 2. Row No.1, was where the Emergency Exit Door was situated, so no invalids etc there then, as dictated by Health & Safety.

The flight took off 10 minutes late but got to Alicante about 10 minutes ahead of schedule, a tail wind did the trick. We of course had assistance all the way through to collect our Luggage (2 cases) which our assistant took off of the Carousel for us and just as we were about to leave the Arrivals Hall. A man showing a card with our names upon started to head towards us, this was our Special Taxi man, (Hooray for special taxi men everywhere).We followed him down one flight in the lift to where our Taxi was parked, where I was then wheeled into the Taxi and anchored in place, there's nothing worse than an unanchored paraplegic flying about in the back of your taxi, now is there? He packed our cases, Maureen sat adjacent to me and we enjoyed our hour's journey to the Hotel Venus in Benidorm.

Upon arrival at the Hotel we checked in at Reception and the staff showed us to our room, bringing our cases with them. The room was on the same level as the Concierge/Reception and was a mere 40 yards away. We were told that the catering staff had laid on a buffet down in the Dining Room should we so wish. We did not bother as it was a little late in the day for us to eat, it was 10p.m. We unpacked a few items, freshened up and went through, following the sound of singing, to the Bar Lounge, where a pretty good male singer was performing. We settled in to some comfortable chairs and had a drink to refresh our taste buds and quench our thirst. We stayed in the Lounge until the singer had finished at about 11:30p.m.and then headed to bed. It had been a good, tiring and very interesting day. We had made it on Holiday without too many hitches, Yippee!!!!

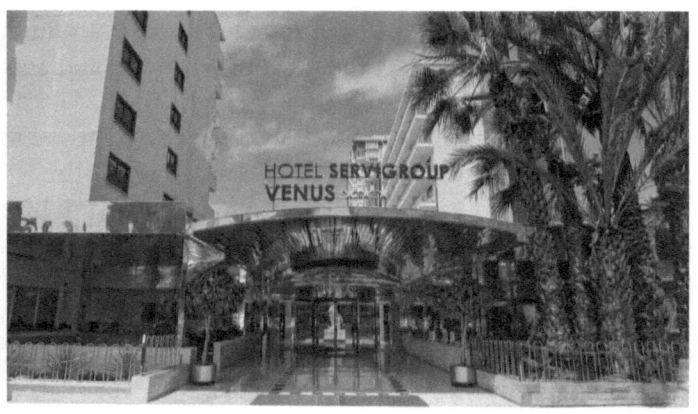

In the morning after a decent nights sleep and directly after our wonderful and extremely varied breakfast we headed up to the Reception area, as we had ordered and already paid for a Double Mobility Scooter for us both, for the duration of the Holiday, i.e. 10 Days. This was scheduled to arrive at 12 noon. However one had already been delivered at 09:30, we took charge of the keys and went to look for this double scooter. My goodness, what a load of old rubbish it was. I tried to drive it a few yards but it was like, what I would imagine driving a Chieftain Tank would be like. It was heavy in fact far too heavy for my one good arm to steer safely. The machine was likened by a passer-by as a relic and one she had refused the day before. We talked to Gill Robinson our "Guest Services" contact and she spent the next hour trying to sort something out for us. Gill told us to call back at about 5:30 p.m. and she said she would have it sorted for then. When we arrived back at the rendezvous as requested Gill said that a single scooter was awaiting us, she gave us the keys and told us the Scooter Number and where exactly it was parked in the parking zone outside the front of the Hotel. We hopped on board and took it for a quick spin around the block. All seemed okay and certainly better than the "Chieftain", with that we went to get ready for our Evening meal and look forward to whatever artiste was entertaining us this evening. The entertainment was first rate, a sort of Matt Monro style. We really enjoyed his renditions he finished by 23:30 hrs.

This is good as it allows hotel patrons to get to sleep at a reasonable hour.

Directly after Breakfast we went out onto the Sunbathing Terrace to take in the Sun's rays and enjoy having the wonderful hot sun on our bodies. I sat reading whilst Maureen went down to the pool for a dip, where she stayed for about an hour, when she came back we had a coffee and sat a for a little time until whilst Maureen fully dried off and the coffee consumed, not a bad coffee either for Spain. We went back to our room to get ready for a ride down to the "Prom", well ride for me unfortunately Maureen had to walk. I asked her whether we should hire another Scooter for her, "I'll think about it" was the answer. After a good run up and down the prom and a stop for the famous and time consuming people watching and perusing the Sand sculptures that are producing by their artists' daily. Some of which are kept in good condition for many weeks, by spraying with water to help keep them cemented solid, but with daily loving touches as well.

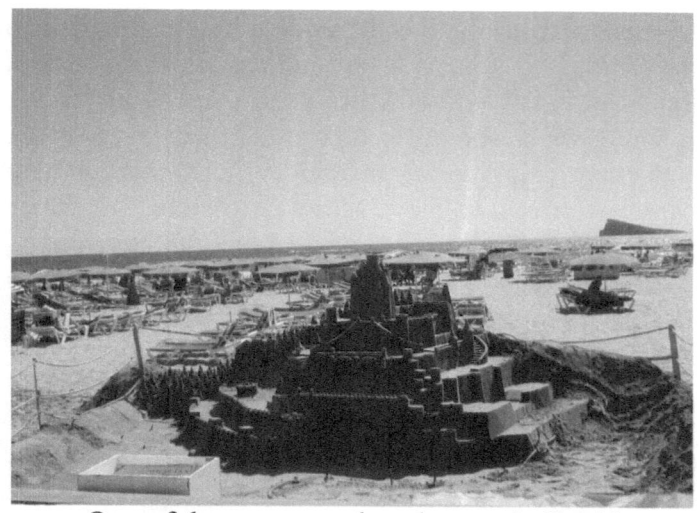
e.g. One of the many sand sculptures in Benidorm

It was now time to call for a light lunch and a drink. Today we went in to one of the many café/bars along the promenade. I found it very awkward gaining access to this particular café but as always, where there is a will there is a way, so no problems but in the end, we put this café on our reserve list of places to frequent, just in case we did not find anywhere better. We finished and started to make our way back to the Hotel when the slight knocking that I had heard on the way down to the front, got louder. Right Maureen let us go straight to Amiga 24 the Scooter Hire Company, which was situated just about 200 yards after our Hotel. We called in to see them, told the man about the noise, to which he said take your pick of another one then. We selected another double, No! that one is broken, How about that double over there, No that is also awaiting some maintenance. Goodness know why these were on their forecourt if they were duds, but I suspect that he did not want us to take one as he could get more money off of the next Hirer, these being doubles and we only returned a single. Even though we had paid for a Double, and in advance. The one we got this time was just fine so we kept it for the remainder of our Holiday. It was time to head back towards the Hotel, we looked in one or two shops on the way then called at "The Meeting Point" for a Beer and a cup of Coffee, guess which one I had. We only stayed for hour whilst chatting and noiseying at other patrons. Then back up the road a little further to the Venus and the scooter park, which is undercover at the front of the Hotel with plenty of parking spaces and power points in which you could re-charge your Scooters. We got dressed and went the Restaurant for our Evening meal.

We had chicken for our main meal, afterwards I decided that I would walk through to the lift. This was a distance of roughly 20 yards, when I reached to doorway, which had sensor controlled curved perspex doors I proceeded to slowly walk through them, this was towards one side of these doors and what became quickly apparent was that I was out of the sensor range. The doors began to close which I saw out of the corner of my right eye. I put my hand against the edge of this moving door, this I hoped would send the necessary signal to the control unit that something was in the way of its smooth passage. The door did not respond to this contact by me and continued on its journey, when it finally reached my right side it still continued and I went over onto my left. I fell like a *"Giant Redwood"* being axed by a lumberjack. I fell straight as a dye onto my left shoulder, arm, & hip. Not the best of feelings I can tell you!. The Restaurant Manager and some of the male members of Staff came to my rescue, asked how I felt and helped me to get up. The manager said "You must not linger when leaving the Restaurant as accidents like this can happen. I sat in my wheelchair for the onwards journey back up stairs. *"Shaked but not Stirred"*. Maureen pushed me outside to feel the evening air, where we lingered for half an hour, taking in the sounds, light and smells of the night. It was then time for our Evenings entertainment and according to the Entertainments Board it was a Shaking Stevens tribute act, probably" The following afternoon we got chatting to this old guy from up Newcastle- upon-Tyne way. I started talking about Medical Travel Insurance and how much it was. This man who said that he had loads wrong with him including Liver & Lung problems, diabetes and high blood pressure and was awaiting the results of some x-rays on the aforementioned Lungs. The man said that he did not bother with Insurance as he always carried enough money to get himself home. Wow! Can you believe that there are still travelers today that think that way. This guy was basically saying that he had enough money to buy an emergency flight ticket back home. I told him about our experience in Turkey and the approximate cost of Hospitalization and repatriation, he gulped and went into deep thought and then went on his way. We never saw him again, maybe he bought his emergency ticket and left for home. Then Gill the customer service lady came looking for us to enquire as to my health and was I injured at all. I had a painful left side and hip from the impact, a few of the ribs felt sore and maybe damaged but no great problem. I asked her to check that the necessary Accident Book report had been made, she confirmed that they incident was on CCTV and that she had reviewed what had happened and that it would not happen again. Well at least not whilst I was there on Holiday!

The rest of our Holiday went off very smoothly and without any further incidental or accidental distractions. The weather was superb everyday that we were there and at the end of the Holiday we were transferred professionally back to the Airport and taken straight up to our flight check-in desk. We were asked to sit nearby whilst there sent for an Assistant to take us through to the Police control and x-ray section and the through to the departure lounge. Then we were asked to wait in a certain area until the departure call time when a further assistant would collect us to take us through to get on the plane. This was done as stated, and once on the plane, we were seated ready for the smooth and on time take-off. The journey back to Manchester was good, once there and with all the other passengers alighted. We were taken off and went through to usual of Custom & Police checks then taken for our Luggage, where yet the same Airport assist guy, that helped us off of the plane, was ready to help with the luggage. We then went through to the Meet & greet area where Michael & Jon were waiting to take us back to good old Sheffield, where we arrived at 11p.m. A long day for us weary travellers, but that's what you have to put up with if you want trips to the Sun!

CHAPTER 18 / Day 465

TUESDAY September 29th 2015

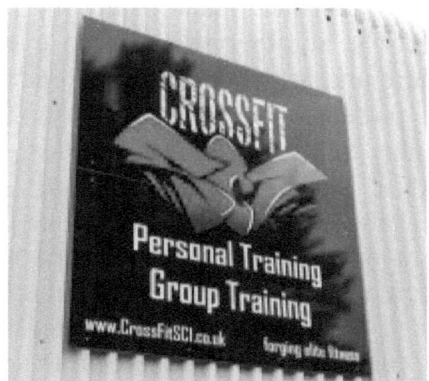

This is Crossfit SC1 in Sheffield, look it up!

This was the Assessment day for the Volunteer Participants in this new type of training. The Neurological Physiotherapy Coach who was running this 8 weeks Course was Gavin Church but he had limited spaces on this course. So the ones lucky enough to be on this Hallam University Sponsored Crossfit course were pioneers on behalf of other Stroke Survivors.

On this first day, Maureen joined me to equally find out about what would happen and with whom, and after all it was only for an hour or there about. On arrival at the Gymnasium, which was an industrial unit on an Industrial Estate. Which surprised us a little as we expected to see the standard type of building. You know all clean lines with many pieces of new electrical exercising equipment...........No not here!

This was a new type of Gym.

Upon entry to this building which was about 25/30 yards square with a floor covering over the obvious concrete base was fairly empty in appearance, that is until you started to assess it with a keener eye. Above to the left of the entrance was a seating area with steps at the far end, where members could relax before or after their workouts with a coffee, or other drinks, that were made available. Below this balcony was the Office the Kitchen and Ladies & Gents toilets/changing rooms. Near to the bottom of the steps were a selection of large aerobic balls and many different weights of what we called medicine balls. Along the right hand side wall was the area within which Gavin kept the vast array of Kettle bells, these ranged from about 5kgs upto 40kgs. Down on the back wall area there were lots of Dumb bells from 3kgs up to 25kgs or there about. There was also a few Bar bells about and a good range of weights to fit these, towering over this area was a Metal frame which was about 12 feet high and the full width of the room. This frame was used for various exercises including chin-ups, pull ups etc.

We all had to walk the twenty yards or so to an allotted square shaped wooden box, These would be our seats for all of our training sessions with Gavin.(These were stored on the bottom left hand corner of this Gym and stacked upon each other). At this first session, as with all the forthcoming 16 sessions (8 weeks on both Tuesday & Thursday), the participants had their weights taken along with their blood pressure to make certain that we had no obvious problems, and were capable of taking part in these exerting exercises. The six of us there had non of the health issues so we continued to do some light exercises to assess our ability to stand stable and hold and raise weights. These were only light weights for this session but would increase in time. There were 5 men and one woman in the group of varying ages from about 36 to 74 years, but all over us were fighting to improve from our strokes residual affects. The first thing you do after having your B.P. taken was just sit on your allocated box and rock your knees from side to side, this was to get you feeling the floor better by re-activating the side-foot nerve sensors. Then we had to stand up and doing the same or similar movements. i.e. Rocking, he then added in twisting the trunk to face the same way as the knees whilst keeping your balance, a total pivot of about 170 degrees. This for me was not easy to attain all the time and sometimes I just fell back into the sitting position. We had a small break whilst Gavin brought us all a either a kettle bell or a dumbbell. Only light weights, My starting weight was 3kgs, the exercise was: place the weight down by your feet then stand straight upright " Squat down pick up the weight in both hands or on hand in my case, stand up straight and pump the weight up to full arm extension, then sit. Place the weight on the floor, Squat, pick up weight push up to full height with your arm, sit back down. On this first day we only did 10 of these, but it was enough for now!

Emma came the day after to work on my arm and re-vitalize my achy body! I was practicing more walking in the Kitchen whilst trying to not walk like a crab (i.e. semi-sideways) You do this by rotating your hips whilst you throw your leg forward, something that is easier when you do not have the control on movement that you would like. However, this is not good as I have to teach my body that the way to walk is to just let your legs swing through with a natural movement and place them just forward of the previously placed foot, therefore moving forward with both legs not just forward with one and matched up with the other. My brain finds this very hard to do at times, but it has to be done and eventually will become the norm!

October 7th Should have been my first day of the Newly organized indoor sports at the Old Rectory, Handsworth, Sheffield as organized by the Stroke Association. This was something that I was really looking forward to trying out these indoor sports Boccia, carpet bowls, maybe T.T. and various others. Unfortunately the Stroke Association who were co-ordinating the community transport to get everyone there failed to reach fruition so unless you could arrange your own transport then "Tough luck". It was too far to travel, cost wise, to pay for our own taxi's for each occasion that this was to take place so I did not bother going. Lots of Survivors did go, the ones who had family to take them there or lived near enough to use taxis. Lucky people! Maybe arranged for my side of the City next time. I do hope so!

I just need to point out to all Survivors reading this book, you are already on the right pathway to even better recovery.   <u>YOU ARE THE PRO-ACTIVE PROPLE</u>!

For every one pro-active type there are at least 1000 more non-re-active types just sat at home awaiting the Services or their Families to do everything for them, rather than attempting to help themselves. The fighters are the real survivors! Just keep up your good and very hard fight!

On my next trip to see Gavin, we started as before after the B.P check warming up the side foot receptors then stand to get the balance active again. We did a few Dumb bell lifts, I started as before with a 3 Kilogram weight then after I had lifted this above my head a dozen times Gavin said could you manage a little heavier weight, yes why not I said! The next Dumb bell was 5 kgs. So we did a dozen lifts with these as well, we took a 5 minute break, to allow us to get our breath back and relax the muscles. We were then re-positioned, our boxes in a line facing the right side wall. This exercise was to walk to the wall, do 15 push ups then walk back to your box then pick your weight up from the floor to full arm extension above your head and then back to the floor 15 times. Next do the same routine but instead of 15 you now do just 9 times, push ups and dumb bell lifts. Then the same again but instead of 9 do just 6 this time. When complete you will have done 30 reps of other. You are timed to completion on this occasion!

October 7$^{th.}$ Should have been my first day of the Newly organized indoor sports at the Old Rectory, Handsworth, Sheffield as organized by the Stroke Association. This was something that I was really looking forward to trying out these indoor sports Boccia, carpet bowls, maybe T.T. and various others.

Unfortunately the Stroke Association who was co-coordinating the community transport to get everyone there failed to reach fruition so unless you could arrange your own transport then "Tough luck". It was too far to travel, cost wise, to pay for our own taxi's for each occasion that this was to take place so I did not bother going. Lots of Survivors did go, the ones who had family to take them there or lived near enough to use taxis. Lucky people! Maybe the Asssociation will arrange this event for my side of the City next time. I do hope so! During the next few weeks I went to Crossfit twice weekly, the exercises got harder and with heavier weights but we all loved it and surprised and surpassed our selves. Rachel Young, Gavin's boss from Hallam University came down to see what we were being asked to do and was amazed at how Stroke Victims could do what they were doing, it really did open her eyes. Lucy Annandale also came down to see us and get some ideas for her Stroke Classes. Gavin's next set of exercises/ circuit training consisted of from sitting on your box squat pick up weight lift high above head back to squat touch floor with weight (repeat 21 times) walk to Metal Framework hold onto ring attached by a canvass strap to upper crossbar lean back fully (roughly 60 degrees) then pull back up. (repeat 21 times). Then back to box for 30 seconds then walk to wall do 21 arm/hand pushups, back to box for 30 seconds. Repeat the above but only 15 reps this time and then same again but only 9 reps. A grand total of 45 reps for each action. You will be timed so speed is very much part of these exercises. It is surprising just how much you can improve on your earliest times. You also do timed walks to & fro to a 10 metre point whilst carrying a weight. (Dumb bell or Kettle bell or M. Ball) on other occasions, not easy for me but Gavin did assist by holding my left arm for support. All these exercises were increased in intensity by upping the weights of the Kettle bells etc almost every time we went. We all managed remarkably well considering our slight deficiencies; it's a good job that all our brains could assess and judge these little alterations in our new work plans.

Abstract.

In the UK up to 73% of stroke survivors fall within the first year. Those who have falls resulting in a hip fracture within the first six months are more likely to die. Ambulatory stroke survivors present with poor balance, weakness, sensory impairment and loss of motor coordination resulting in a falls risk. Intervention through exercise and strength training can be inconsistent and there appears to be a degree of variability in the application of functional strength training. Crossfit style training uses constantly varied functional movements performed at a high intensity addressing all aspects of fitness and utilising all three energy systems. It has a strong community and social network and is used by athletes in various sports because of its foundation of general physical preparedness.

The aim of this study was to investigate if an eight week intervention based on the principles of Crossfit is feasible as an intervention for improving balance and gait in ambulatory stroke survivors

A twice weekly intervention over eight weeks delivered to six participants. Changes were measured using a mixed methods approach incorporating the performance orientated mobility assessment (POMA) outcome measure combined with a focus group in the last week. Data analysis for the POMA used the paired students t-test. Analysis of the focus group was devised from using themes in previous research and analysed using open and closed coding, thematic analysis and pattern identification.

Five participants completed the study and all individuals demonstrated significant improvement using the students t-test ($P=0.05$) with POMA scores apart form the one participant who achieved the ceiling for the measure. Findings from the focus group were positive and supported the findings from current literature.

Of the five participants who completed the study three were considered high falls risk and two were low. On completion four were low falls risk and one was moderate falls risk. The focus group themes were around enjoyment, individualisation, challenging and supportive over conventional exercise experiences and improvement in self and externally observed functional aspects of daily living.

Crossfit appears to be a feasible intervention for reducing falls risk in individuals six months post stroke. Participants enjoy the safe, challenging, individualised and effectiveness of the intervention in comparison to previous exercise experiences. Larger scale studies, more sensitive functional related outcome measures and further investigations into the mechanisms for improvements need to be considered.

gavin.church@nhs.net

CHAPTER 19 / Day 484

TUESDAY OCTOBER 18th 2015

On Sunday 18th October 2015 whilst riding my Leo Scooter to the Hillsborough shops I suddenly noticed that I had got an object stuck to my front offside tyre, I stopped and Maureen pulled off this object, which just happened to by an ear-ring the sort with a back stud which had pierced my tyre, but with being small and I had very good tread on the tyres did not think anymore of it for the next few minutes at least. Going along the pavement on Bradfield Road the Scooter started pulling a little to one side. We carried on the Precinct shops, when Maureen called in Fulton's for some milk, I started to have a look at my tyres and found that the offending front off-side tyre was pretty much flat. We did not bother to do much more shopping and tried to get home with the Wheel in tact. Because we had really good tread on these tyres, we managed to get back home and said that I would have to get it fixed by talking to the Shop where we had bought it, the following day. Monday morning a telephoned the shop and they gave me their repair centre telephone number and told me that it was £80 call out charge plus cost of parts. We rang the repair centre and arranged for them to come to do the repair. We they eventually came he quickly took the tyre off inserted an inner tube. Re-inflated the tyre and charged us £80 plus £10.78 for the part fitted. That is not the sort of Ear-ring that I like, very expensive and cheap looking! When we saw Michael & Jon on Sunday we confirmed with them that they were still up for a trip to Benidorm the following June, yes we would love to go with you for a week. I said that I would sort out the Flights with our Samantha who manages the Kanoo office in Sheffield. (The Ex-American Express Company) also the Hotel & airport transfers direct with the Venus Hotel in Benidorm. Monday morning I phoned my lovely God-daughter/Niece and discussed what we would like her to do and that being Alicante flights from East Midlands Airport for 7/8 nights with special Airport Assist for me plus 3 other travellers and a Wheelchair. Sam phoned back later with our Options. We settled on an 9 day/8 Night Holiday, so it was the go on a Tuesday come back on a Wednesday, with the assist and wheelchair booked in the Premium seated area. More leg room for us all, which was needed for my passage in and out of the seats and Mike & Jon for their longer legs.

The following morning (Day 492) I telephoned Gill Robinson at the Venus to book rooms for all four of us, we agreed on Rooms 8005 & 8006 as good ones for us, 8005 was the one we had checked out in September when we stayed there. I had agreed that I could manage that room without any special adaption's because it had a specific configuration. Gill told us the room prices for half board and printed them off for us. The verbal booking was made and confirmation was received via email later. She also sorted out the special Taxi that I would need, because I would be with my Wheelchair on Holiday, just for the longer walks that I would need to do! This too was booked and this had to be paid for up front. Not cheap but needed and after all it would get us to the Hotel a lot quicker than the usual transfer transport. We shall look forward to this Holiday, even if it is a long time between now and actually setting foot in the warmth of Spain in June. The Schools were on their Autumn break and so was the Crossfit Gym. A whole week off, Mmm shall have to do some weights at home and I don't think the odd can of beer will cut the Mustard. Otherwise I will turn back to being just a Jellybean, so crack on Rog with loads of squats, walking and one arm press-ups against the wall. The Press-ups I did against various walls both indoor & outdoor, most of the walking was done up and down the length of the Kitchen with the odd trip up & down the stairs and the Squats I did with the use of my Railing outside the back door. I also managed a little walking without any form of assist equipment, A First I believe and I was thrilled that I could do this with no physio present at all! Most of the time down at Crossfit there was just four of us, sometimes five and just occasionally six. The four of us namely Keith a Basketball Coach, Shaami a charming alround athlete, me and Marine an ex-netball player, who could lift any weight that Gavin gave her to lift, he also started showing us how to professionally do a dead lift by dropping the body whilst firing your arm up to full height extension. Marine was a natural at it, I used to pull her leg about being in training for the ordinary Olympics in Rio let alone the Disability ones that followed the able bodied. Of the other two that were on this course, One of these guys worked **part time** so only came down to the Gym **part time**. Number six was ill/unfit to participate for almost all of this course, but made it there a few times. Sunday 15th November came and so did Mike & Jon, they took us out to Dobbies Garden Centre, an excellent place to come for any Christmas trees or Decorations you may need plus loads of ideas and quite a few good shops. Whilst we were there we got looking at some small

Mobility Scooters as I needed one to able to use on Public Transport (i.e. One metre long maximum and only 4mph top speed were allowed) I agreed to buy a Pride GoGo Elite Traveller LX with 3 months free Insurance and a few other perquisites' to go with this. But only after both Jon and myself had a little practice, up and down the Shopping Arcade that we were in and just outside the Scooter shop. It was agreed that this Scooter would be delivered on Wednesday the 18th and that they would adapt my Leo Scooter so that it would become very difficult to puncture in the future by filling the tyres with a solution that kept them from going flat unless a huge chunk of tyre got ripped off, torn away or blow off in a violent gale, accidentally. On Tuesday 17th, I had an appointment with Dr. Ali Ali at the Royal Hallamshire Hospital for 11:15hrs. We arrived promptly as always and were directed to the waiting area about 50 yards down the corridor adjacent to his "Surgery for the day" room number ? whatever it was! We only waited about 15 minutes and my wife & I were called in to see Dr.Ali. I was expecting a botox injection(s), but Dr. Ali said that he was passing me on to a Doctor that was better at this and was the head of the "Spastic Clinic" at the Northern General, Doctor Singh who would be in touch with regards to my Spasticity and the Botox injection(s). Dr. Ali thought that I would soon hear from Dr. Singh with an appointment. I thought, I bet that will be Easter time then!...............Oh ye of little faith!.

    Wednesday came and my New "Supertram/ Omnibus sized Scooter" arrived as planned and the Tyres on my "Leo" were done as agreed. No more problems with standard punctures, but there was less give in the tyres so therefore not quite as comfortable a ride, but okay! Nor was the New GoGo Elite which had the small wheels and solid tyres. I would have to be extra careful when travelling on uneven ground or where any hazardous material may be left i.e. this mainly relates to supermarkets who dump stuff all over the shop until told to "Shift it" by their bosses, customers can't get around!

Thursday 26th November. Mrs.T's birthday, and the last of the Scheduled sessions with Gavin at the Crossfit Gym. We did the long circuit today starting from the Box. The weights had gone up again but there were no complaints from the four of us that were in attendance, we all enjoyed it there. First pick up weight, floor to ceiling lifts then to the wall for pull ups, then back to the box rest 20 seconds. Then to wall for the push ups back to the box. This first circuit was of 21 repetitions 2nd was of 15 rep. and the 3rd was of 9 reps. So the new total was 45of each and as I said the Dumb bell, kettle bell weight had gone up, in my case it was roughly 3 times the first weights I used, and we all did this Routine in about half of our original time. Which were at the old weights and lesser repetitions Gavin was right in that he selected the right people for this Section of his Study course towards his MSc. We had to go back just one more time to the Gym and this was for Gavin's wife to assess us has she had done before we started this course, this was to take place on the 3rd December. We each arrived back at the Crossfit for assessment on this date and were all asked for our opinions of the course along with any concerns that we may have had. This was not so much our Assessment but the courses, Gavin & his wife, who often assisted Gavin, just needed our feedback to add to their reports. We all appeared to sing from the same Song Sheet, that was we all really enjoyed the experience and we asked if Gavin would be doing any more of these courses, and if so "Then pick us in" yes please was the cry. This has not happened as yet but maybe shortly, who knows!

CHAPTER 20 / Day 526

Sunday November 29th 2015

At 10a.m. on this last Sunday in November I had arranged with the Local bus company for me to take my Scooter Test, this Test was to see if I was capable in being able to embark & disembark with my new one metre long Scooter on & off a bus. Although the Test was always done on a bus, the resultant License would cover me for both Buses & Supertrams, should I pass. This morning I drove down to the nominated bus stop, the lady with whom I had arranged this test arrived driving her double Decker bus and parked up. She came and told me what she expected me to do and unfolded and lay down the ramp for me to drive up into the bus. Gently driving onto the bus with no spare space around me, I now knew why they only allowed Scooters up to 1 metre long,. Longer ones would not be able to manoeuvre in this tight space. After turning to the right I could see that I was adjacent to the "Parking Area" The idea was to drive past and reverse into it,

That was really awkward not being able to see backwards or even over my shoulder (a thick short neck does not allow this movement too well at all) but after 3 or 4 minutes I made it. The thing is, for safety reasons, you must park with your back to the driver at all times. Getting off was easy it was just a case of full left lock back a little and then same again, down the ramp and all done. Whilst I was disembarking Michelle the driver was writing out my pass License which has a lifetime of 3 years after which you just reapply, as long as you have the same Scooter.

On the 4th December my wife came with me to the Northern General Hospital and to the Spinal Injuries centre which is where the Spastics centre is located, to see Dr Singh who was to take over my Spastic problem. Once inside, we were told by Reception to go through to Doctor Singh's waiting Area. We were called in to his surgery roughly 15 minutes later. Dr Singh was waiting there, as was Alison Clarke from the F.E.S. Clinic who was directed by the Doctor as to where to inject the Spastic releasing Botox into my Arm. When this was over they said that a new appointment would be quickly forthcoming for some physiotherapy to assist the injection to do its job. Also they would get onto Orthotics to fix me up with a brace for my Wrist & Hand. You got the impression that these appointments would happen quite quickly!.......Mmm?

CHAPTER 21 / Day 542

Tuesday 15th December 2015

THE JOLLY SEASON!

Denise & Bill took Maureen and myself to the City Hall on the 15th December 2015 Day 542. to see & hear the most Wonderful Grimsthorpe Brass Band (Made extra Famous in the film "Brassed off") for their Christmas Concert. It's the first time that we had been to a Brass band concert and thought that after a couple of tunes we would get "brassed off" as well! Well we didn't, we had a really enjoyable evening and hopefully get to go again in 2016. Denise had organised some superb seats near the front but equally close to an entrance/exit door. I was taken in by wheelchair, transferred to my seat okay and the said chair was parked just behind the place where we sat. After the concert was over they took us home with time to watch the evenings episode of "Coronation Street" that is on catch-up TV. We went to bed rather happier than we were when we went out.

On Wednesday the day after the Concert, Paul from the Stroke Association was having a meeting at H.A.S.A. a local sports centre where our Denise is the Manager, and is only about 200 yards from home or 300 by pathway through the Park. Both Maureen & myself decided to pop in and see what he had to say. Paul had little to say and nobody else turned up, so what a waste, pity!?

The day after Maureen had a Christmas dinner with some friends from her walking group whilst I went, as usual, to Lucy's Gym for a good Pre-Christmas workout, create a space for the necessary food, that I would have to endure, Poor old Rog He! he!

On the 21st was the Table Tennis Clubs sort of Christmas knockout competition up at Shiregreen, so I didn't last long then did I! However my friend and driver Neil did well, I believe he was the Runner-up. It was an entertaining evening with free drinks and Pizza on the Club. Neil ran me home for about 10:30, a long night for me, but hey! I don't have to get up early in the morning, so why mention it!

Emma came about 1pm the day after and worked on my much resistant arm, I'll be glad the day when we can manage to find my start button for the said arm. My brain is constantly telling it to get a move on, but alas there appears to be a blockage with my electrical impulse nerve serving my left arm and also I have a similar situation with my leg, but this is not quite as isolated as my arm. Come on chaps listen to my grey cells, please!

Christmas Day arrived with a bacon & mushroom butty, (my favourite meal each week) Maureen always treats me with this for my Sunday breakfast or in this case Christmas brunch. After it was, *"Open the pressies time"*. I'm just a big daft kid at times..........Lovely!

We were collected later and taken up to Michael & Jon's for our Christmas Lunch, It was as always wonderful, the Wine and Jon's superb food, cooked to perfection as one would expect from one so accomplished in culinary skills. Whether they are meats or vegetables or desserts, all were enjoyed immensely, it's just a shame that my appetite these days, is just not up to large meals. We had a coffee and a few After eight mints before adjourning to the Lounge to watch the Telly! We did not stay with them too long and asked Michael to take us home at about six p.m. That way they could relax without us cramping their style and we could all settle down in our own lounges to watch the rest of the Televised evenings entertainment. Restful & Happy.......

On New Year's Eve we went with Bill & Denise to the Cinema to watch "Heart of the Sea" which was a non Captain Ahab version of Moby Dick. The Story was all about a New England. USA whaling community and a Captain who got enthralled by the Big Whale. It is a really good film and quite spell binding throughout. Then it was back home for a quiet drink before "Lights out".

THERE ENDETH 2015   ROLL ON 2016
Yippee!

CHAPTER 22 / Day 559

Thursday 1st January 2016

2016

On 8th January one of the Doctors from the Surgery where my records were kept, rang and asked me whether I would go back on Statins for a trial period of two months to help get my Cholesterol a little lower than it was. This I did a whole 8 weeks then I had to organise a nurse to come and take a blood sample. After 3 calls about this, the nurse phoned and made arrangements to call. On the due date & time she arrived and blood was extracted. We rang the surgery the following week and then the week after, we then got a text to say. "You will need to rearrange do this again in 3 months time". The surgery you see is situated on a hill which is inconvenient for my abilities to attend so we ask them to call.

About a month later we dropped in a form that I needed a Doctor to sign, It was just about being able to claim financial assistance back, for my private Physiotherapy, from the Health care scheme that I pay into each Month. He wouldn't sign it because he had not seen me, so I could not go to the Surgery and they would not visit me, so stale mate or so we thought. Maureen went up to the G.P's practice to see another Doctor for herself and mentioned the situation to her. She said that she would sign the letter and send it off the Health Care Scheme. This she did, and we are most grateful to her, even though you have to pay, to the Practice, for this privilege.

We went up to the Northern General to the FES Clinic to see Alison Clarke on the 20th and the 22nd January. The first visit was as a follow up on the Injections given to me by Dr. Singh, just to see whether I thought they had worked. They had helped to ease the arm off a little but was still very tight, whenever I moved around doing any sort of movement. My second visit was to return the FES Control unit for my leg as it was uncomfortable to use, with its strong pulsations when walking. I would use a foot up splint instead. We were back up at the Northern yet again on the 26th Jan. this time to Orthotics to see Connor Moreton; the appointment was about getting a splint for my left arm. Connor checked my arm/hand and made the decision to get me a ???? I will have to order one for you it should take about 3 weeks to arrive.. I received the Splint 6 weeks later on the 3rd March 2016. I took this splint home but we found it very awkward to get on my arm, but we have persevered! Today 29th April I went back the Northern General Hospital to see Dr Singh. He gave me some more Botox injections in my left arm and told me to carry on with my stretching exercises and working with Emma. He wants me to go back in 3 months on a follow up visit!

As per 2015 I volunteered to assist Emma with the University MSc. Course as before, just a body for the Physiotherapists taking the course to work on. I went a total of 6 times, which included their Assessment day. I do so enjoy helping out on this Course!

After the problem I had in getting a G.P. to sign the Health Care Scheme letter, I decided that I should change to another Practice, one where I could actually get into. I did this on the 30th March.   Emma brought me a leg splint to try out and if okay, If could keep it, it does and I have! The following week on the 14th April she brought me a new type of Splint for my arm. It was a different design from the one from the Northern but similar in some ways. It seems to work better, however its only on loan for 2 weeks or I could buy it for £200 plus. A bit costly, but never say never as the Rehab Assistants always like to say.

Most of the time now it is: Gym twice weekly or out occasionally with Alan & Pauline to the Devonshire Cat Pub or My mate Pete's calls, for a chat or I have Emma around for a Physio Session. The rest of this year I am looking forward to continuing our Family visits and being able to get around on my Scooter and indeed on foot, if mainly around, but occasionally for short spells in Hillsborough Park. We are really looking forward to our June Holiday to Benidorm with Michael & Jon, Jon has not been there before so he is even more keen than we are to his break from work and a new experience. I hope that we may even be able to get away for another break later in the Year, as I shall hit 70 in December, 70 by the way is the new 50!

CHAPTER 23

Emotions & Feelings Part 2
(Chapters 9 to 22)

The whole of the time that I was in either of the Hospitals or in the Rehabilitation Centre, a Time scale of:
AHU Hastanasi (Turkey)   2 Weeks and one day
Royal Hallamshire Hospital 5 Weeks and two days
Oak Lane Rehabilitation Centre. 5 Weeks and two days.
I had no moments of emotional weakness!,
It was just a case of do as they ask, enjoy and utilize what was good: the Physiotherapy, some of the Staff, and some of the food.
What was especially good was the camaraderie I had with some of the other Patients/Inmates. Especially George Cockayne! (I wonder what ever happened to him?)
Work hard and try to get home as soon as possible. On the day of departure some of the Staff, the ones that were good to me or even liked me, came to wish me good luck, I even got a kiss on the cheek off of the Head Physiotherapist, **yes It was a women**, *but by that stage I had given up caring about who was what sex! I just needed to be home and start to progress by myself, but obviously with the great help of Maureen plus the home care package team, Physio's and their Rehab.assistants plus the occasional Occupational Therapists. Some of them talk to you as if you are a piece of meat i.e.* ***I know best****! You do as you are told etc. Not good!*

After a few weeks I managed to change their attitude enough for us to work properly together from there on. They were good lasses

Really, but stuck in there own world doing what they had always done, and that was to take control of the whole situation. Some folk just do not realize that encouragement is better than a big stick. I know that the big stick is necessary with some lazy patients but not all, and that includes me.

Once Home I started to weaken a little when I could see that Maureen was definitely struggling with all the chores she had to and wanted to do, but alas she wasn't 35 any longer and it was taking its toll on her strength. She was absolutely marvelous cleaning the house, making the beds,(I was sleeping on a hospital bed in our Lounge at this time) cooking, washing, ironing, **pointing the brickwork, scrubbing the walls, painting the grass etc. etc.** *She also had to help transfer me from one place to another by the use of a Rotunda, which for Maureen weighed a ton to manoeuvre about the house, this was to help me in my placements such as bed to commode, commode the Lounge chair, Lounge chair to dining room chair, or to the bed at the end of the day. A man would find this exhausting let alone a woman of mature years.*

It really/was only when I saw Maureen under this greatest of pressure of work, that I got weepy, because most of the time I could not do a bloody thing about it! Oh I wish! It is supposed to be my job to look after her when we get older, which we have. Maureen always tells me that my job is **"To get better".** *So I do my best to oblige.*

The one thing emotionally that has changed is the fact that when I see or hear something really good or very nice or courageous I find it hard to control the corners of my mouth from dropping and the eyes from watering. Even tough cookies crumble when under attack from the Goodies!

CHAPTER 24

<u>Stroke Recovery Stages</u> (as I see it)

1) Surviving the first few days.
2) Recognising that you have had a Stroke and the first attempted Movement.
3) Cognitive Recovery: are you talking sense, do you see what others can see, can you hear okay.
4) Do you know what happened to you and where, but certainly not why. (you may never know this)
5) Become pragmatic and start to come to Terms with what you may well be stuck with.
6) When you have come to Terms with the Stroke you may start to ask Questions. i.e. How long will my recovery take, no correct answer can be given! What happened within my body? You will find out that it is not just your face that can drop but all the organs within your body cavity, this is why incontinence can be evident from day one, but may not be!
7) You will start to think of ways that you can assist your recovery. Whilst ever you are in the Hospitals or Rehabilitation Centres, always work hard at all forms of energy sapping or mind blowing exercises, especially the ones that "I can't do that" keep trying until you succeed and then try even harder.
8) When you get home and can do small amounts of controlled movement start with helping with the washing up, after you have washed, dressed and had breakfast that is. After this it is time to

move on to Jigsaws, Crosswords & Puzzles or reading or using a computer or tablet etc
9) Then onto Activities outside the home. Walking on your pathways. i.e. to your gate and back, but not until you are physically and mentally ready. Or if you are capable and have a large wheeled wheelchair, push yourself off of your property for a bit of fresh air with different views. The same four walls everyday can send you a little stir crazy.
10) When you have made sufficient improvement within yourself you may fancy going to a gym or swimming, as these both give you great exercise but greater mind power and give you a lot more confidence about your own abilities and knowledge about how far there is to go.

When you are at this stage then you are well on your way to the better life. Good luck and work hard, as it is hard work!

MY FALLS & STUMBLES

As it so happens I do not fall about much, I put this down to the fact that I have played Sport all my life and for the last 40 years played League Table Tennis. This in itself gives you good balance, but when you coach as well then you get to know more about how this movement with balance works.

I digress:

1) I lost balance when walking past my settee about February 2015, roughly five months after I had got home.

2) Same as first, A misbalance about a month later.

3) In April I was stood in my lounge when I lost balance again but thought "That's alright I'm close to a wall" wrong I was about 3-3.5 feet away from the wall and door frame,, which I hit with such a wallop. My lefthand side of my back was sore for about a week.

4) Easter Monday 2015 Whilst walking along my back pathway towards the gates. I stopped to look at the plants. Probably turned too quickly and sat on a pebbled area, yet again no injury!

5) September 2015 This happened when an Automatic door failed to sense me and started to close and knocked me sideways, I fell like I had been shot, well I did go with a bang! Ribs hurt for a few weeks after that one.

6) Boxing Day 2015 Heading to the stairs at 10p.m. I thought that I heard my wife setting the Burglary Alarm so I tried rushing a little. Silly billy I stumbled and went down straight legged and head first. Result a slight bruise to my face and a few sore ribs.

7) Late April 2016 the community transport called to take me to Pond's Forge. However they were a little early so I was rushing to get to the garage to get my Scooter and because of such I took my eye off the ball and stumbled into my garage wall and the concrete planter at its base, No damage as it so happened, so I carried onto the Gym as planned.

These are my only falls or stumbles to date and each one has been caused by a lack of concentration, so keep alert at all times or at least until you can move really well to try and counteract these mishaps,.

CASE HISTORIES

No.1

Mr W. A regular cyclist who, on this fateful day, decided to have a pedal out to Rother Valley Country Park a distance of 4/5 miles from his home. Just to get some exercise, fresh air and because he enjoyed cycling. Whilst propelling himself around the Park, he gradually started to feel a little unwell. So he set off for home, a wise decision, No doubt! Mr.W continued to feel a little off during the rest of the day but thought nothing of it and went to bed. The following morning he was still under the weather so made contact with his G.P. who asked him to pop in and see him later that morning. The Doctor ran a few quick tests and suggested to Mr.W. that he had suffered a Stroke! This was met with some surprise as by the now, Patient. He was sent to Hospital for an MRI scan to confirm his diagnosis which it did..................... Conclusion!........ Strokes are not always highlighted by the tingling in the arm or and side, the dropped corner of the mouth, the slurred speech, the affected vision, the lifeless limbs or any other things that you may know or heave heard of from friends, the TV ads or the G.P.'s surgery waiting room. Stroke's can occur without any tell tale signs but I will bet that you don't feel too good at the time that they happen. Mr.W still has problems differentiating between red & Green, as in Traffic Light colours and numbers in General, he probably suffers from Daltonism, but has not confirmed this. Therefore with this problem he has not been able to take a disable driving course or test because of these issues and maybe will never be able as it seems to be an ongoing situation. He still suffers from right arm pain daily!

No.2

Mrs.P. Just felt unwell went to her G.P, and was told she had probably had a stroke..................Simple as! She is making a fantastic recovery, but like all survivors, she still has issues!

No.3

Mr.B. You know straight away that this Gentleman has had a stroke, he has great problems being able just to talk about them, and it is as though his Brain cannot find which Dictionary to use. On some occasions finding the words needed are not a problem, but on others, well that's different! This man has to push his wife around in a wheelchair as she suffers from internal organ frailties and severe Gout which cannot be easily eased by the normal Allopurinol tablets as these interfere with other medications. So she has to grin and bare most of this pain. The man's had a Cholesterol based Stroke and he has to assist his wife.....I do not know how he does it. When you've had a Stroke it should be you who gets the help. Mr.B and his wife go on Holidays abroad such as the Canaries and Cruises, but the latter is just a bit too much as they have trouble trying to get off the boat when visiting other Ports. That is a big pull for Cruise ships, but it is just a little bit too much of a strain to get wheelchair users off of them. At 70, life does not always get easier with age!

No.4

Ms.S. Had an epileptic fit 20 years ago and as a consequence of this suffered a stroke. She was in her early thirty's with a three year old daughter when this happened to her. First she was taken to the Hallamshire Hospital and then later transferred to the Northern General Hospital to stabilize her condition. Can you imagine just how devastated she must have been! A thirty four years old with a 3 year old, and a Stroke. I bet she thought life was all but over! However she found what can only be described as massive strength and the ultimate desire to do her very best for her daughter. She summoned up "***STROKE STRENGTH***", this is the inner core that all survivors have to find, just to cope with life let alone all the other major differences that have occurred within their own bodies. Ms S did not get the NHS back –up that all of today's' survivors get. Such as a Rehabilitation Centre and 13 weeks of home Physiotherapy or the Assessment and Rehabilitation Centre that is ARC. Or assistance with referrals for F.E.S (Functional Electronic Stimulation) or any Botox injections to assist relaxation of the arm/hand.

When you know what you want to say and you just cannot get the words out, this what Ms.S has put up with this all the time. When I was asking her about her residual stroke affects and she was trying to tell me what they are and she could not get the words out. I said that's fine you have answered my questions by not being able to speak about them…….enough said. If having one Stroke is not debilitating enough, then having another on 15 years down the line is an extra massive kick in the guts, but this is what happened, so its once more she had to send for the *"STROKE STRENGTH",*

This Lady has had a very tough time of things but she is still fighting for improvements in her body, brain and limbs. Maybe one day a light will shine in her direction and not just on a stroke victim who is fortunate enough to recover without too many ongoing problems as some of these lucky people just do not realize that for some, things take time and if not in twenty years then maybe by twenty five years, lets hope so. Good Luck Ms.S.

No.5

Mr. F.

This Gent, who is blind in one eye, had his Stroke at the age of 78, he was alone at home and was found on the Floor of his bathroom after a wait of 4/5 hours. He had struggled throughout this period of infirmity, trying to get up by using all and any of the fixtures and fittings that were within his range of movement, no luck there then, so he had to wait for reinforcements to arrive. This came with the appearance of his niece's partner, who organized the ambulance to take him off to the Hospital, where he stayed for 9 weeks before being sent the same rehabilitation centre as myself He stayed for a further 8 weeks, before he was considered safe enough to be allowed home. This gentleman is a true fighter, he lives alone with very little family help, because there is not a lot of them too help. He battles on daily and is a great inspiration to us all. It was a good thing that he always kept himself fit by doing lots of walking, Especially out on the hills, moors and valleys of

North Derbyshire. Not many people of his age, not having the luck of the writer of having plenty of family living in the same area of the City, is absolutely amazing. I think we all hope that should we ever finish up in similar situation to him, that we have at least half of his strength & resilience to carry on the same as him.

No.6

Two years ago during the early part of July Mr.T was sat in his conservatory when began feeling unwell, he called to his wife who was in the garden, by the time that she had got back to see what was the matter, he had slid off of his seat onto the floor. He was having his Stroke and was discharging his waste in all directions and was perspiring most profusely. His wife rang for an emergency Doctor who arrived 5 hours later, good job that it was an emergency or he could have been there for days! The doctor checked him out and gave him an injection to stop the vomiting but nothing for the other end. What most people do not realize about strokes is that ALL your internal organs drop down. It is pretty much the same as when you die, you empty your bowels, not in all cases but this also happened in my case. Later the same day whilst <u>still</u> on the floor where it happened, his wife said that he had better try to make his way upstairs otherwise he would be staying the night in situ. He crawled up to bed over the next 45 minutes to warmth and safety. The day after his wife sent for another Doctor who when attending to Mr.T suggested that he thought he had had a Stroke , sent for an ambulance who then whisked him off to the Royal Hallamshire Hospital for assessment and a stay, when confirmed that a Stroke was the correct diagnoses. Whatever medical help was received by this Gentleman must have worked well as very few residual problems are not apparent.

He has made a remarkable recovery, maybe this was because of his Army Training or the amount of Sport that he played or any other of his multitude of activities, but this Gents fitness was definitely a contributory factor to take into account, in his recovery.

No.7

Mr.D A year ago at work this Electrician started feeling unwell, his son with whom he worked said "I think that you are you having stroke" nonsense he thought, I shall be fine after a rest.

He went home and to bed "to sleep it off,(as you do) However he did not sleep it off, the following day the he was just the same. The day after it was decided that he must go to the "Drop in Centre" to see what they had to say about his condition. A Doctor ran some test and within 30 minutes he was in the Royal Hallamshire Hospital. Another life saved! Mr.D's main problem he has been left with is that he has lost a lot of his peripheral vision. No doubt that all the people I have talked to whilst gathering information about their Case Histories are not telling me everything. However, having a Stroke is just the start of a whole new way of life and all so often it is a totally different way than before the Stroke.

No.8

Mr.J. Suffered a Stroke almost 3 years ago and is now making significant progress since his arrival at the Stroke Gym rum by Lucy Annandale at Pond's Forge Sports Centre in the Heart of Sheffield. John was out in the fields on his Tractor when the stroke took place. He managed to stop the machine but then fell out on to the field itself. Fortunately a neighbour noticed that there had not been any movement of the Tractor for a while and enquired off of Mr. J's wife, if all was okay. They rushed out to the field to check and found him beside his Daily Workhorse, the tractor. They rang for the Services and was taken to the Royal Hallamshire Hospital, after many weeks he was transferred to Oak Lane Rehab Centre, A place that he hated, not that many liked that place but it did do a little good with the minimal amount of Physio that they could give to each Patient. If only they could have afforded more Physio's then I am sure that all patients would have improved quicker. When he was allowed home he had spent six months since that fateful day on his tractor.

Since he got home and with the help of very good NHS therapists, he has progressed. His affected hand/arm have been able to recover their movement and strength but he still has a way to go yet with his leg strength and control…..good luck!

No.9

Mr.K Two and a half years ago he had felt unwell at work, the next day it had not sorted itself out and now his heart rate was racing and somewhat erratic, he went off to Hospital and it was decided that to correct this they would fit him with a Pacemaker. When this was fitted and switched on it sent a blood clot straight to his Cerebellum, the area of the brain that controls your voluntary movements, this caused him to have a Stroke. This resulted in not being able to walk or swallow and was fed via a tube. His eyes were also affected as was and is his balance and was confined to a wheelchair for household movement for quite a while. However this guy is of true Yorkshire grit & determination and with the Physio's help and a walking aid, in the form of a stick, soon managed to get up and start to walk a little. His walking is now good and he has no feeding problems now. He is doing very well with his fitness and strength but as yet cannot return to work

No.10

Mr.R Was 57 when he had his Stroke over 8 years ago, he drove to Leeds and back when he felt, should we say "a bit off". He arrived home safely, then decided to go for a game of Golf at this point he started to feel a little woozy and was making strange noises, the left side of his face started to droop. It was realized that he was having a Stroke and 99 was rang. The ambulance arrived and off to the Northern General for assessment. Once assessed, he was moved to the Royal Hallamshire Hospital, where they have a Specialist Stroke Unit, this would be his home for the next 16 weeks.

Up until that day he and his wife had spent a full and active social life and both were still working, this finished with the Stroke. This was a huge disappointment to Mr.R as he enjoyed his work at the same Company for 30 years, but alas no more working, golfing, socializing with his mates of fund raising for a Charity, which is close to his heart. Prior to the Stroke he had experienced sessions of "Pins and Needles" down his right arm and frequently dropped items. His G.P. thought that this may be Carpel Tunnel Syndrome. (It's a shame that it wasn't)

The stroke left him with little or no use in his left arm/hand and very little leg movement with no foot up movement. He also had vision impairment and found it hard to swallow and talk. The Stroke had taken this proud man's Independence as it left him unable to do anything for himself. That of course was 8 years ago, today he can walk a few steps with his trusty quad stick, but needs full assistance in all other matters. He finds this very frustrating and sometimes, just sometimes, feels a little depressed. He tried the disabled driving test but discovered that it was just a little tough, at this stage in his recovery.

No.11

Ms G   At 45, I was moseying along in my life. I had a job that I loved and worked very hard at. I loved my partner, family and friends and enjoyed travelling and spending time with them. I thought I was taking care of my health by not smoking, not drinking to excess, eating very healthily and doing lots of exercise. One morning I got up to go about my day, not realising that everything was about to change. I had a headache that steadily worsened but I was used to having migraines so just carried on as normal. I had visual disturbance unlike my usual migraines but didn't think too much of it. As I was walking out of the back door from the kitchen to drive to work, I realised that I was falling to the floor backwards. We had been redecorating so there were boxes of decorating equipment and paint tins on the floor. I was aware of thinking "this is going to hurt". The next thing I knew, I was on the kitchen floor. I couldn't get up, but didn't realise that I couldn't move the left side of my body. I spend some time wriggling around trying to pull myself along with my right hand. My next awareness was laying half out of the kitchen with my head and shoulders on the drive and my legs in the kitchen. A leaflet distributor found me and offered help. He got me up but of course I couldn't stand or walk so went down again. He went next door to find help. When my neighbour came, she realised straight away that I had had a stroke and phoned an ambulance and my partner, who phoned my family in different parts of the country. I wasn't long at A&E but was taken by ambulance again to the stroke unit at another hospital. After various scans and tests I was put in a bed on the stroke ward. Coming to, I found my family, partner and best friend lined up along the bed – it was such a relief to have them there. For three days the doctors didn't know whether I would survive. It also seemed I would need surgery to remove a piece of my skull in order to relieve pressure from the swelling caused by the stroke.

After several weeks on the hyper-acute and acute stroke wards I was transferred to a stroke rehabilitation unit where I was given daily physiotherapy. After several weeks there I returned home. It was great to be home but also very frightening as I had still had no use of my left arm and hand, and was only just able to take steps with a walking aid (tripod). Banisters and hand bars were fitted to the staircase and toilet which helped me to get around a bit.

Now, two years later I go for weekly physiotherapy, which I pay for myself, every therapy class that is available, and do all the exercises, I am given several times a day. I still have no functional use of my left arm or hand. I am beginning to manage walking without a stick but it will still need a lot more work before I can throw the stick off a high cliff! I am determined to make a full recovery and will keep working until I achieve this and get back to work. For now I still need carers to help me get washed and dressed. My family, partner and friends have been wonderful and so supportive, as have all the hospital staff, physiotherapists, etc. I would not be where I am without them, although I still have a long way to go before I achieve my goal.

No.12

Mr.P Almost 2 years ago whilst at our Caravan in Lincolnshire I began feeling a little unwell and starting to develop right-sided weakness. The following morning my wife noticed that my face gad drooped and suspected the worst. The paramedics were called, they ran some tests and took me off to Scunthorpe General Hospital. However at this stage I was still capable of walking in to the Hospital, who took me through to a ward, where they did some more tests. The following morning when I woke I found that the Stroke had hit! I could not move my right side one iota, and my speech was slurred! I was later transferred to the Royal Hallamshire Hospital in Sheffield and taken to one of their Specialist Stroke

Wards, where I stayed for the next 4 weeks. Slowly with the care & help of the Nursing staff and the Physiotherapists movement started to return. Firstly my fingers started to move followed closely by my toes and then my arm and lastly my leg. All very slowly but they were actually moving. Whatever exercises I was asked to do **I did.** At the end of the four weeks I was transferred to Oak Lane Rehabilitation Centre for another couple of weeks before being discharged to home. All the Physiotherapy that I had received to date had been wonderful but a lot more would not have gone amiss. I was able to walk a little by the end of may two weeks with them just as the Physio. had promised! I managed to pass a driving test to prove that I was capable of doing so without killing anybody, especially ME. I now go to regular exercise classes aimed at stroke survivors and Lucy the referral coach is extremely adept at getting the best out of us and to help us improve in so many ways. I too like many others have had to retire from my job and accept that life has changed for ever. However by meeting similar survivors at the Gym and being able to discuss our problems, you feel that bit better after every trip there. I am one of the Lucky ones as EVERY DAY IS A BONUS.

As for myself:

It is almost two years since my outlook on life had to change. I pay for Physiotherapy and other forms of activity, such as Ponds Forge Gym or if we need to get out we pay for the use of the Community Transport. I am Mentally and physically strong (on my right hand side, that is) My left arm currently has about 2% use in it, but we are working continuously for its improvement, My left leg for most of the time feels like carrying a 4 stone side of bacon around. Although I can feel the movements and the contact sensations that I have with it, I even have a little control over such. The leg is getting better and I feel that it is currently at about 13% of its usefulness. Small improvements are being made and I shall forge forward with all effort to get more general control along with more muscle for its placements. The section called "My Heroes" are the people who have and are assisting in this process and without whom, I would have and would be struggling. For this reason I consider myself very lucky to have met some of my fellow Pond's Forge Gym users, as these are all ***Real Heroes***

At times Stroke patients will often smell odours that nobody else can smell, whether these are real or not I don't know, but I have heard this from numerous survivors, I for one certainly do! Also you can be just sat watching the TV for instance, when you think that you have seen something out of the corner of your eye. You may well have, but this too is just one of the quirks that can happen, after a Stroke.

These few Cases are from the pro-active survivors, ones that do something about getting an improvement in their daily lives. However for every proactive type there are 1000 that do nothing positive at all.

The ones that sit at home waiting for the never arriving miracle!

These Historical Cases are just a synopsis of some of my Stroke Friends, experiences. These friends are Male & Female with ages ranging from their 40's to their 80's. All are different, all are fighters and all are very much worthy causes. Some with obvious signs of a Stroke, I am a prime example of this with my left arm always fixed across my body when walking or doing any form of activity and my slow and deliberate gait with my Walking Aid. Others not so obvious, fingers that are not working properly, eyes that are losing their ability to see well or at all, hearing that gets less efficient, voice that has trouble communicating, Mind control over all these plus not joining up ALL THE DOTS!. And a thousand other problems that that may come to light later.

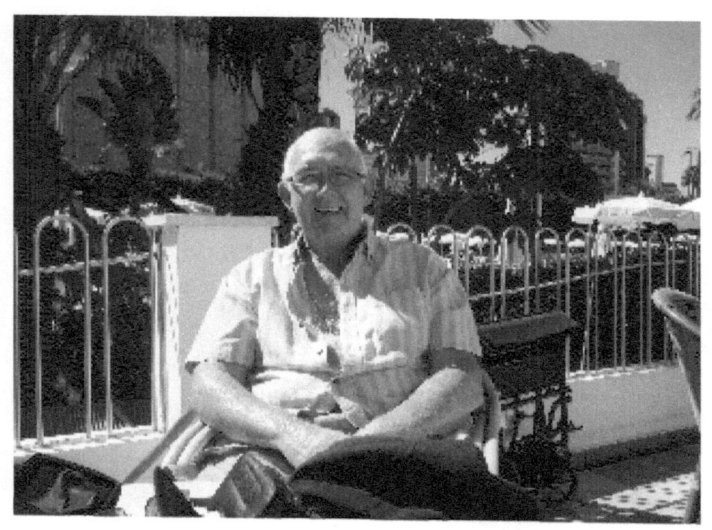

ABOUT THE AUTHOR:

I am Roger Turner and am currently 69 years of age and live with my wife Maureen in the northern area of Sheffield, South Yorkshire. U.K. We live a good life, although illnesses to us both has slowed us down. Our family lives mainly in Sheffield with Our Son, Daughter and one of our four Grandchildren, 27 year old Jack, all living within a mile. We live in a modest semi-detached house adjacent to a Park, where I spend time taking in the air whilst gadding about on my Mobility Scooter.

I was born and reared on a Council housing estate in the east of the City and went to the local school. I became a cub scout for a couple of years at a local Parish, which is where one of my school teachers played the Church organ, he talked me and a few of my classmates into being a Choirboys, which again for me lasted only about 2 years.

We moved across the City to private housing when I was 11. I did however continue my schooling at the old school because of my swimming potential.

I did not pass my 11+ (A compulsory National examination that determined whether you was clever enough to go to Grammar School or not.) simply because the idea of *"Daily Homework"* really deterred me, as I was a hyper-active child, and wanted to play sport 24/7. I represented my School at Swimming. Football, Cricket & Gymnastics. After the 11+ exam, all my classmates who were ranked above me, and 11 who were ranked below me, all passed to go off to Grammar Schools. (*What a dumbbell was I*)?

Proven by the fact that, although I was a City Champion swimmer at 9 years of age. I never actually attained the necessary improvement to do it again. Oh I won plenty of district championships but no more City wide ones. The School teams of which I was a part, won many Trophies year after year. But all these sports never led to any long term success for me. The only other thing I won whilst still Schooling was the North of England Junior Softball Championships, a team which I captained and represented the local Mormon mission.

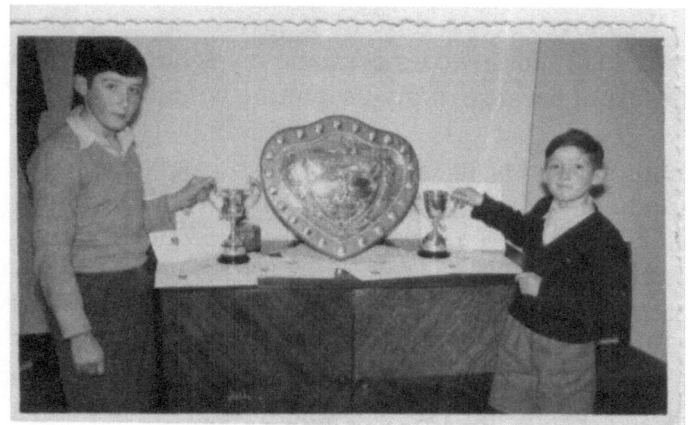

With my big brother Alan (a National swimming Champion.)

My friends and I met some Mormon Elders, in a local park one day, and they got us into playing this North American Sport, we took to it like ducks to water, probably because it is quite similar to Rounder's, and we all played that at some point in our School life. With me being the most extravert of all us kids, was appointed Captain.

When I left School I was fortunate to become an apprentice electrician, but that on lasted 13 weeks as the company ran short of work and I along with others got laid-off. I spent the next 4 years in the Grocery trade and attained the position of under-manager. I passed 13 trade exams whilst with the Co-op.

My spare time, as always was Sport, I played Football for the Sheffield Ambulance Service, dad worked for them. I cycled and hiked at lot and did a spot of Caving/Pot Holing & Rock-climbing. I also joined the Gymnastic Club based at the local youth club, where I also played badminton. I then joined the "Hillsborough

Boys Club" where I played Table Tennis with the Sheffield Junior Team, a sport I really enjoyed but when you don't win many games, probably because of their high standard of play; you call it a day and move on.

I was then asked to represent the Club in the Yorkshire Boys Clubs Swimming Championships; I was fortunate to win the Backstroke Final and was Runner-up in the Butterfly Final. I am not too sure how I ever managed to do all this sport to any decent level, as I had <u>smoked</u> from being very young when on that Council Estate, until I decided to "give up" at the ripe old age of 48. I smoked the odd fag from about 8 years of age, cadging and procuring from wherever and however. From about 15 years old I was on about 22 cigs a day, i.e. 8 x 20 packs a week, for the next 33 years. Packing up was the second best decision of my Life………..The first is obviously my Wife.

*It appears that I Captained a lot of teams etc, Well that's what happens when you have a **big mouth**!*

At the age of Nineteen, I applied for and was appointed to the job of an Office clerk, at Engineering Company in the City's East-end, a company for whom I worked for the next 42 years. It was a specialist Company and in time, I became firstly, the General Office manager, Sales Manager and then Purchase Manager. This job initially started as just buying Stores supplies for the shop floor. Later, because it looked like the Company may fold, due to competitors cheap imports', It was decided that I should go to China and to source new suppliers, ones that could provide us with quality cheap products. This I did until I took an early retirement at the age of

62, just a short while after I had had my one and only T.I.A. (a mini-stroke.)

The Managing Director and I had negotiations on my possible retirement once that I had returned to work. This was not something that I had thought about, I thought that I would carry on for a lot more years, he thanked me for my support and the service given to the company and offered me a package that I could not refuse.

I went home and discussed the deal with my wife, Maureen thought that the deal was good and more than we could have expected, so we agreed that I should retire, now that I was fit again. I took me a couple of days to bring colleagues up to date with what was happening. I then cleared my desk, cleared my computer and desk drawers of any personal stuff and after having had the discussion with my wife.

Retired..................Simple as!

The main sport in my Adult life began in 1970 when with some friends we started to play Table Tennis on a borrowed Table. The owners of which were the then local League Champions, and having watched them a few times, got the bit between our teeth and started a Club. I, amongst others within the club, became Qualified Coach and indeed I became the Leagues Coach in a very short few months. i.e. *Thrown in at the deep-end.* When I started to Coach the youth of Sheffield I was somewhat naïve, but with the assistance of others, got the kids playing a good standard of T.T. Within the next two years Sheffield Junior and Cadet teams' dominated the Yorkshire Leagues in which they played, and won all the Titles & Honours available.

The club we started won the League championship Once and many other Divisional Championships over the following years' we became known as the most prominent coaching club in the League. Provided the City & County with many players, both male, female, Cadet, Junior, Senior and Veteran.

The complete Club. until it folded in 2010

I met my wife through T.T. Her husband Ben ran the Sheffield Inter-City Junior teams whom I coached. A man, who was a great friend and colleague and who died at the young age of 40 years.

Ben had became a member of our Club along with his young daughter, Denise, I could see straight away her potential. I told Ben that if he and Denise wished I could start to coach her. She had previously played a little at another Club, as is where the start to her playing career had started. She took to the sport most proficiently and played not only for our club in the League, but also with a couple of years, Sheffield Ladies.

After about a year I was lucky enough to start dating Maureen, and the year after we got engaged, whilst taking our first Holiday together, in Gibraltar. During the Christmas holiday of the same year, 1980, we got married. (It was a bit of a rush, but well worth it!)

We have had and will continue to have, God willing, a great marriage and life together. We have had loads of really good holidays both abroad and in the U.K. We shall continue to do so.

To try to put down one's thoughts about one's life is never easy. Should I have just skimmed over my history or given an even more in depth statement, I don't know I will leave that to you to decide.

<u>I hope I have got it about right!   If not please forgive the twitterings of an old Fart!!!!!!!!!</u>

MY HEROES
Aka Possible the world's greatest Life-support team

In case the book beats me to the end I would like to dedicate my Story to the one person who endured the latter part of my life the hardest but with the most love. My Wife **Maureen,** she has put her own health and strength into jeopardy into giving me the utmost Love and Help possible and tendering to my every want and need. A person with whom I am so pleased to have shared my life with. With all my Love Rog.xxxxxxx

I also would like to thank my Family, Denise & Bill, Michael & Jonathan along with Grandchildren Jack, Annabell & William & my big Brother Alan and his wife Pauline for their great help and encouragement. Also our great friends, Maureen & George, from across the road and Peter Muscroft my long term buddy and sporting colleague.

Not forgetting the Specialists that have helped, firstly the NHS Doctor's, nurses and physio's at the "Royal Hallamshire" and the nurses and physio's at Oak Lane Rehab Centre. The NHS home physiotherapy that I received along with some good home Occupational Therapy, especially from Ruben Steel. Also Alan Mowforth@ARC the Nether Edge out-patient Rehab Centre.

I would really like the Thank whole-heartedly my personal private **Physiotherapist**, **Emma Richards** for the mental & physical assistance given to me, that has got me in to the position of the ongoing strength that I have today. **THANKS EMMA**

Also Many thanks to Gavin Church and Lucy Annandale and assistant Rebecca for their "Special Gym" work outs. Cheers Guys

And Thanks to all the people who have help to create this my Story and that have added input in support of me.
E & OE

SPECIAL ACKNOWLEDGEMENTS

Many thanks go to Maureen my very special wife for all her love and encouragement and daily proof reading, in the production of this, My Story.

Thanks go to Denise & Bill for their help and the Trips to York, Various Garden Centre's, The Theatre and Cinema and their useful purchases made to help me.

Thanks also to Michael & Jon for your great attention to us and the many meals out and the little trips, including Matlock Bath, that we have had and the many helpful purchases made. Most of all thanks for asking us to go on Holiday with them this Summer. Cheers lads!

We would like to thank my Brother and his wife Pauline for the extra care, love and help that we have been paid since day one of my Stroke. I also want to thank Alan for helping find a Publishers and for verbal distribution of my book, on my behalf. Thanks!

Thanks to all my Case History friends for their Stories

Also massive thanks to Emma Richards my Physiotherapist for Proof reading and medical input, along with the writing of the Foreword.

My wife and I would particularly like to thank our good neighbours Maureen & George for all the little things they do for us like: Putting our Rubbish bins out, and bringing them backing, in all weathers January to December. Bringing various items in from the shops including the Saturday papers or Freshly laid eggs or whatever we may fancy. It saves my Wife & I a lot of hassle, especially at Weekends. They are always buying little things but they will not ever let us pay. If ever you need a guard dog or a special envoy, go out and get a Maureen, there great! I have two, one at home and one over the Road. They are the best protection a man can have, so don't delay go and get yours now! My wife is My Rock, my Vault, my Panic Room,

My **"SANCTUARY" XX** and obviously my Life

Places that I have Visited and Sites that I have seen

I have been very lucky throughout my life and have been most fortunate to say the least in being able to travel to many of the Worlds Beautiful places. I have seen "The Valley of the Kings, the mighty Aswan Dam, the magnificent Abu Simbel and the Temples of Karnak and Luxor and sailed the majestic Nile. I have been punted by Gondola down the Grand Canal in Venice, I have been to Hong Kong and looked down onto Kowloon Harbour from the heights of Victoria. I have walked on the Great Wall of China, visit the Forbidden City (aka the Imperial Palace) the Temple of Heaven and the Summer Palace, all in or around Beijing. I have not only seen the Niagara Falls but flown over them in a Helicopter, sailed up to them on the Maid of the Mist and walked behind them. I have stood on the glass floor on the Viewing Gallery of the C.N. Tower at 1300ft. looking down onto Toronto, and not only been in a Cable car ride to the Top of, and partly inside the "ROCK" that is Gibraltar, but all around the this marvellous out post. We have Toured all around Vienna by open Landau, holidayed in beautiful Paris, ascended the Eiffel Tower, seen the Mona Lisa at the Louvre and admired the view of the beautifully built basilica of Sacre Coeur on Montmartre., not forgetting the Cathedral of Notre Dame. Visited a Spice Plantation in India. Been enchanted by the Wonderful Ruins of Ephesus and Cotton Castles at Pammukale and not forgetting the Blue Mosque and Hagia Sophia Mosque and the Grand Bazaar in Istanbul, all in Turkey. I have been to the top of Columbus's Column in Barcelona. Also I have visited many other Countries and a vast amount of Greek & Spanish Islands. We have owned a Static Caravan situated on the East coast and a couple of Touring Caravan's which we have towed around the UK.

*Lucky extremely "**LUCKY**"*

I DO NOT REGRET ALL THE THINGS I HAVE DONE IN MY LIFE AND I WILL NOT SURRENDER TO WHAT IS IN STORE!

A FOOTNOTE

To all Stroke survivors: whether your stroke was Cholesterol based or Hemorrhagic based or for any other reason, fight like you have never fought and do it continuously and without thinking. FIGHT! Use all forms of help that you can find and or become a member of these forms of help.

<u>Never ever think of giving up.</u>

Put your hand up for everything and anything that may help with your recovery. The more you volunteer for projects, courses, classes, or other helpful possibilities, the more you will get <u>rewarded</u>. You do get better almost every day, if only you could monitor these miniscule improvements.

<u>**ONWARD & UPWARD**</u>
   After all it was ***<u>Just a Stroke of Bad Luck!</u>***

<u>**Always believe in the power of positive thought!**</u>
   I have had a great life and done lots of things and visited loads of Country's and seen lots of sites and experienced lots of new and sometimes strange occurrences.   All have been *GREAT!* *EVEN SOME OF THE STUFF I HAD TO EAT IN SOME OF THE DISTANT VILLAGES IN CHINA'S INTERIOR,* (When on business there) .. i.e. Food you do not want to even think about. Don't forget in China, if it moves you can eat it!

You may well think that life is not good at the moment, but believe me it really is better than the *ALTERNATIVE*.

As my old belated Mother-in-law would often say "STILL BREATHING"

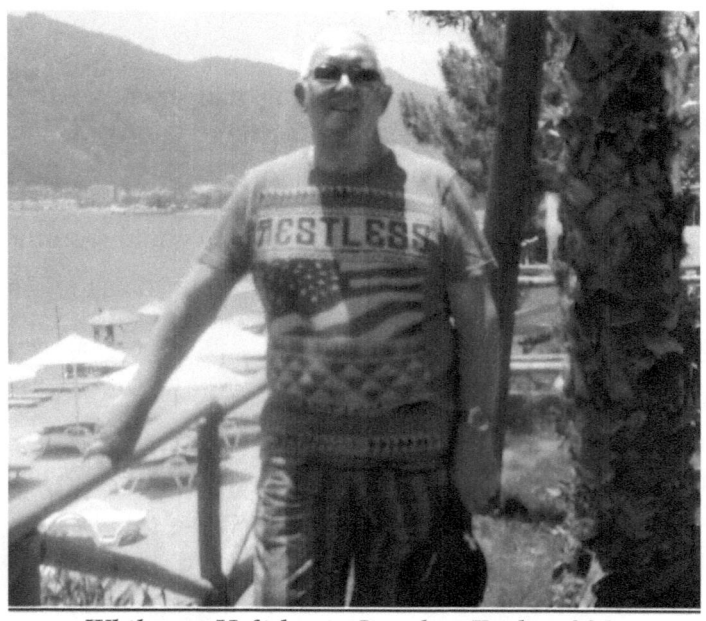

Whilst on Holiday in Icmeler, Turkey 2014

www.ingramcontent.com/pod-product-compliance
Lightning Source LLC
Chambersburg PA
CBHW020652220526
45464CB00001B/408